POULTRY DISEASES : CAUSES, SYMPTOMS & TREATMENTS

Dr. Narender Kumar Vyas

AMIGA PRESS INC.

DELHI (INDIA)

AMIGA PRESS INC.
H.O.: 28-A, Indra Park, Chander Nagar
Delhi-110051 (India)
Tel.: 011-22504028, +91-98736-57000
E-mail: amigapub@gmail.com
Website : www.amigapress.co.in

This edition is published by Amiga Press Inc.

ISBN: 978-93- 87295-04- 9

First Published 2019

Printed and bound by Amiga Press Inc. New Delhi-India

Preface

With millions of poultry farms around the world, the business of producing poultry and eggs is becoming more concentrated and accelerated in the recent years especially with the technological innovation and modern brooding equipment and reduced cost-price compared to the last years.

Poultry diseases are diseases that afflict poultry. The eradication of poultry disease is very important to the poultry industry. Major types of poultry include chicken, turkey, duck, ostrich, cornish game hen, etc.

Poultry can be affected by a variety of diseases and parasites, some of which are endemic to certain types of bird. As highly pathogenic avian influenza H5N1 virus continues to circulate in the world, poultry farm biosecurity and timely reporting of morbidity and mortality among commercial poultry farms. To assess the vulnerability of poultry farms to the introduction and spread of a highly infectious pathogen, such as the currently circulating H5N1 influenza virus.

In general, avian influenza is a disease of birds caused by bird-specific influenza A virus that is not normally transferred to people; however, people in contact with live poultry are at the greatest risk of becoming infected with the virus and this is of particular concern in areas such as southeastern Asia where the disease is endemic in the wild bird population and domestic poultry can become infected. It is possible that the virus could mutate to become highly virulent and infectious in humans and cause an influenza pandemic.

Sincere efforts have been made to insert all pertinent pathological changes in different poultry diseases with the object of making this book of high value to the students at both undergraduate and postgraduate levels in the veterinary colleges.

– Author

Contents

1

Introduction

A good history will often provide clues that will help solve a problem. Get information on the type of bird, age, feed and water source and consumption rate, growth, production, morbidity and mortality, the description of the case, previous problems, vaccination programme, medicine being used etc.

The problems may relate to management, environmental factors, and stress rather than to infection so examine the yard and housing conditions. Is the ventilation adequate? Are ammonia fumes a problem? Is it too hot or too cold? Is the litter wet or is it too dry and dusty? Is the pen too light or too dark? Are there sufficient hours of light for best production? Is the nest area darkened? Are the roosts too high? Do the birds appear comfortable? Chickens can talk and the sounds they make can indicate comfort, hunger, pain, panic, or disease.

EXAMINATION OF LIVE BIRDS

Check the general appearance of the individual or group and try to determine which organ or system is involved in the illness. Note any signs or lesions that might point to a diagnosis, such as small size with poor feathering that suggests infectious stunting (malabsorption syndrome). If the birds show lameness or paralysis, is the lesion in the nervous system, bones, joints, muscles or skin? Some conditions, particularly those affecting locomotion, are easier to diagnose in live birds. Botulism which produces neck paralysis in chickens (leg and wing paralysis are more obvious in turkeys, ducks and pheasants) is an example.

Examine the skin of the head, body and legs for lice and mites, injury (particularly cannibalism), blood, mottling, swellings, anemia, cyanosis, or dermatitis. Listen for unusual breathing sounds (snicking, gurgling) and look for gasping or head-shaking that might indicate respiratory distress. Mouth-breathing (panting) is normal in chickens in hot weather. Exudate from nostrils and eyes and dirty feathers also suggest respiratory infection, or if just the eye, ammonia burn, ILTor eyeworm. Examine the droppings for evidence of diarrhea or other abnormalities. Take a blood sample for haematology or serology if indicated.

Necropsy. If a postmortem examination is to be carried out, birds that are representative of the problem in the flock must be selected. If birds have died, both sick and dead birds should be opened. Cull birds will not provide the answer. If the problem is a drop in production, try to find birds that look like they have recently stopped laying. It is important to do both an external and internal examination and to follow a specific routine to avoid missing important lesions.

- CRD - chronic respiratory disease
- IB(V) - infectious bronchitis (virus)
- ND - Newcastle disease AI - avian influenza
- CA(V) - chicken anemia (virus)
- EDS - egg drop syndrome
- IBH - inclusion body hepatitis
- ILT - infectious laryngotracheitis
- IBD - infectious bursal disease.

Live birds may be killed by cervical dislocation except when anemia or respiratory disease is suspected.

1. Examine the head, including the eyes, ears, nostrils, comb, wattles, mouth and beak.

   Infected eyes and conjunctivitis are seen in CRD, sinusitis, Bordetella and Orthobacterium infection, infectious coryza and in ILT, IB and ND.

   Keratoconjunctivitis with central corneal ulcers suggest ammonia burn.

   Swollen sinuses are seen in infectious coryza (Parahaemophilus infection) in chickens, sinusitis (mycoplasma), cryptosporidia and Bordetella infection in turkeys and pheasants. They may also be seen as the result of other infections such as influenza.

   Chronic fowl cholera causes swollen wattles and sinuses in adult chickens.

   Fowl pox causes scabs on the comb, eyelid, and wattle, but must be differentiated from injury. Pox also occurs in turkey, pigeons, doves, canaries and other birds.

If the bird has had its beak trimmed, check for proper healing, overgrowth of the lower beak or over-trimming (cut too short). Injury on the head, neck or breast or back may indicate predators. Dermatitis and scabby or crusty lesions around the mouth and eyes suggest vitamin B deficiency.

2. Cut across the upper beak and back into the sinuses; then through the mandible and down the esophagus into the crop.

   White plaques in the mouth, esophagus, or crop may be caused by capillaria worms, yeast infection (candidiasis, moniliasis), or possibly trichomoniasis or vitamin A deficiency, but most frequently by fowl pox (wet form). White plaques beside the tongue in the mouth are common in hens and turkey breeders and may be caused by mycotoxin or low humidity. Vomitoxin may produce similar lesions in young chickens and turkeys.

   If the crop is enlarged and full, it may be an impacted or a sour crop (pendulous crop). The problem may be caused by excess water intake, defects in the crop itself, partial blockage of the proventriculus or gizzard or Marek's disease. Necrosis of the crop in wild birds is caused by Salmonella infection.

3. *Examine the soft palate and larynx and cut down the trachea.*

   Wet fowl pox lesions are seen on the roof of the mouth, pharynx and larynx.

   Granulation, congestion and mucus in the trachea are seen in CRD, IB, coryza, ILT, Orthobacterium, Bordetella, and E. coli infection, or with dust and ammonia fumes.

   Hemorrhage and blood clots may occur in ILT and in ND or coryza and may cause severe gasping.

   Gapes (gape worms) in pheasants, quail, and other birds is caused by Syngamus infection which also causes gasping. Cyanthastoma cause similar infection in water fowl and tracheal flukes may be found in waterfowl. Tracheal and air sac mites occur in cage birds.

4. *Check the abdomen for lice and mites, and the vent for injury and prolapse of the oviduct.*

   Cut down between the abdomen and the legs and dislocate the hip joints. Peel the skin off the abdomen and breast. Tightly adhering skin and dark tissues indicate dehydration. Remove the breast carefully by cutting through the abdominal muscles, ribs and coracoids.

   At this point, examine the thoracic and abdominal organs, paying particular attention to the air sacs, lungs, and liver. Carefully raise the gizzard and intestines and examine the abdominal air sacs, peritoneum, spleen and the ovary in laying birds. The air sacs are cloudy in respiratory disease such as E. coli infection, Mycoplasma, Aspergillus, IB or early CRD in chickens. If there is also fibrin on the liver and in the pericardial sac, suspect E. coli or Salmonella infection. These lesions in turkeys and other birds might also be due to Chlamydia, or in ducks Anatipestifer infection.

Pneumonia in turkeys is caused by fowl cholera (Pasteurella multocida infection), and the lungs are quite solid. Aspergillosis, ND, AI, E. coli and Ornithobacterium infection can also cause pneumonia. Peritonitis in layers is usually "egg peritonitis" caused by E. coli infection from the oviduct, although acute fowl cholera also causes peritonitis.

White crystals on the heart, liver and other tissues and organs are uric acid crystals (visceral gout) and are caused by hyperuricemia from urate nephrosis secondary to water deprivation, urolithiasis or other kidney disease.

Large blood clots in the abdomen or hemorrhage and hematoma on the liver are the result of trauma or fatty liver hemorrhage syndrome in chickens, or ruptured aorta in turkeys.

Tumors in or on the organs may be Marek's disease, lymphoid leukosis, or other varieties of tumors. Multiple small tumors on the organs and peritoneum in adult hens are metastasis from a carcinoma of the oviduct. This may result in ascites.

Ascites may also result from heart or liver disease or from ingestion of some toxic material. Right ventricular failure occurs most frequently in meat-type chickens after 4 weeks. It occurs secondary to pulmonary hypertension causing right ventricular hypertrophy and valvular insufficiency.

Focal white lesions on the organs may be tumors or they may be tuberculosis or coli-granuloma or, if just on the liver, blackhead. Turkeys, pheasants, and peacocks are all quite susceptible to blackhead; chickens are less susceptible. There are prominent cecal cores in blackhead (Histomoniasis) and occasionally in salmonella infection or coccidiosis.

In chicks, turkeys and waterfowl, examine the lungs and air sac for yellow-white foci or plaques caused by brooder pneumonia (Aspergillosis). Gasping in young birds is a sign of tracheal or bronchial epithelial injury, or obstruction and can be caused by irritating fumes or by infection (often IB plus E. coli or

Aspergillosis). In young chicks, look for an infected navel and for yolk-sac infection or peritonitis (mushy chick, omphalitis) in which the abdomen is swollen, wet, and discoloured, and the yolk-sac is infected (due to E. coli, Salmonella, Staph., Proteus, etc.).

Young birds also die because they don't start to eat (starve-outs) or drink (dehydration). Deaths occur mainly at 3, 4, and 5 days. This may be a management problem (chilling, feed and water not available, etc.) or the chicks/poults may be weak or defective when hatched.

Broiler chickens that die suddenly from sudden death syndrome (dead in good condition) or from heat stroke, or suffocation (piling- up) have congested, edematous lungs, a full digestive tract and congested mottled breast muscle.

5. *Examine the circulatory and immune systems, the heart, pericardial sac, blood, spleen, bursa, thymus, and lymphoid tissue of the thigh and intestine.*

Birds that die from anemia are pale and the blood is watery. With CAV the thymus is small and bone marrow may be pale. Birds that bleed to death (pick-outs, ruptured fatty liver, acute cecal coccidiosis, ruptured aorta, hemorrhagic enteritis in turkeys, etc.) are also pale.

Sulpha poisoning produces anemia and widespread hemorrhage in the tissues. Chicken anemia virus (CAV) produces similar lesions and is the agent responsible for infectious anemia associated with IBH. Lead poisoning may also cause anemia.

To identify anemia from parasites in blood cells (Plasmodium or leukocytozoon in ducks, turkeys and chickens), blood from a live, sick bird must be examined.

IBD (Gumboro disease) is caused by a virus that damages the bursa causing illness in 2-4 week old chickens or in younger chickens destroys part of the immune system, making birds more susceptible to other infections.

Swelling, congestion and hemorrhage with or without focal necrosis in the spleen, liver and lymphoid tissue suggest septicemia (fowl cholera, fowl typhoid, streptococcosis, or erysipelas) or viremia (ND and duck virus enteritis also affect the lymphoid tissue in the intestine).

Marek's disease and lymphoid leukosis produce tumors in lymphoid tissue and organs except for the bursa which is mainly affected by lymphoid leukosis (occasional Marek's lesions may occur in the stroma of the bursa).

Skin leukosis is Marek's disease virus causing viral dermatitis in the feather follicles. At processing this can be confused with scabby hip or other causes of dermatitis. Marek's disease can also cause lymphoid neo-plasia in the skin.

6. *Cut through the proventriculus and remove the digestive tract and liver.*

   Open the proventriculus, gizzard, and small and large intestines to the cloaca. Check the cloaca carefully for evidence of picking injury.

   If hens are not properly beak-trimmed or are too fat, mortality from "pick-out" is common. The whole intestine may be picked out through the cloaca. Prolapse of the vagina (and cloaca) (blow-out) may occur from excess fat or straining, secondary to injury or inflammation. Injury is common in flocks that produce large eggs before they become mature. Examine the digestive tract for lesions and the various kinds of enteritis (hemorrhagic, necrotic, ulcerative, etc.), parasites (tetrameres, roundworms, capillary worms, tapeworms, cecal worms, and coccidia), and gastrointestinal accidents. A large proventriculus in broilers is from lack of fibre in the diet resulting in poor development of the gizzard. A thickened proventriculus sometimes with ulcers or hemorrhage may be Marek's disease or infectious proventriculitis.

   Green staining of the digestive tract is just bile and indicates that the bird is not eating. The liver and spleen may be small (if the bird is thin) and the gallbladder full. Salmonella pullorum (pullorum disease, bacillary white diarrhea) causes enteritis, diarrhea and death in chicks. It has been eradicated in many countries.

   Check the ceca, intestine and liver for lesions of blackhead, TB, coccidiosis or tumor, the liver for other varieties of bacterial, viral or protozoal hepatitis, cholangiohepatitis etc., and the pancreas for tumors.

   A large liver may be lymphoid leukosis or Marek's disease, or it may be caused by bacterial hepatitis (E. coli, campylobacter) or fowl typhoid (Salmonella gallinarum).

   Hepatitis with necrosis and hemorrhage that looks like bacterial (vibrionic) hepatitis may be immune damage to veins (vasculitis) from amyloid.

   A large, yellow liver may be normal fat storage in a laying bird (estrogen stimulation) but layers die from fatty liver hemorrhage syndrome. This occurs when the liver ruptures because it has become fragile due to excess fat and free radical damage from fat.

   A yellow or hemorrhagic liver particularly with focal necrosis may be viral hepatitis (IBH) which is seen in broilers, pigeons, raptors, owls and psittacine (but IBH does not cause infectious anemia).

7. *Examine the testes or ovary and open the oviduct. Shrinking ova indicate illness of 2-7 days' duration or one from which the bird may be recovering. Small, sac-like ova indicate that the bird has been out of lay for a week or more and may be in a molt.*

   Semi-solid (cooked) ova indicate bacterial infection (such as salmonella).

   An impacted oviduct may be secondary to vent-picking, egg-material left in the oviduct, or the bird may be egg-bound. Infection (Mycoplasma, IB, E. coli) can cause salpingitis as well.

   A large or small fluid-filled cyst in the right abdomen beside the cloaca is the cystic remnant of the right oviduct (may be normal, but increased by IBV).

   A drop in production may be related to clinical or subclinical disease (EDS, IB, MG, AE, AI, ND, etc.) or management faults (lack of light, temperature change, lack of water) or nutritional problems etc. Deformed shells suggest management faults, superovulation, EDS, IB and soft shells (higher than 1-2 per cent) calcium or vitamin D3 deficiency.

   A normal-appearing dead bird with an egg in the shell gland, or just laid has likely died from acute hypocalcemia. These birds often have fragile bones (particulary the femur), lack of medullary bone and rib infolding (osteoporosis, osteopenia, osteomalacia).

   Hard (fibrotic) or swollen testes indicate bacterial infection (salmonella).

8. *Examine the kidneys and ureters.*

   Swollen, pale or white spotted kidneys indicate hyperuricemia from urate nephrosis and may be due to lack of water or other kidney disease. Swollen, pale kidneys are also seen in IBH, IBD and fatty liver and kidney disease. Ureters plugged with hard stony material (urolithiasis) indicates a previous low phosphorus diet.

   Swollen kidneys and nephritis may be due to IBV (nephrotrophic strain) or E. coli infection and usually causes death from dehydration. Newcastle's disease causes lympholytic foci in the kidney in pigeons.

9. *Examine the skin, integument, muscles, bones and joints.*

   Emaciation, along with small organs, suggests malnutrition, stunting syndrome, beak injury (poor trimming), peck order (psychological) problems, chronic disease (coccidiosis), bumblefoot or other lameness, or chronic poisoning (lead, insecticide, etc.).

Muscular degeneration due to vitamin E-selenium deficiency can cause lameness, particularly in ducks. Ionophore toxicity causes muscle damage and paralysis in turkeys. Granulomas in the breast muscle are usually a vaccine reaction.

Sarcosporidial cysts produce small, white lesions in the muscle of water fowl.

Examine bones and joints for abnormality and deformity. Angular bone (valgus-varus) deformity of the intertarsal joint is caused by lateral or medial bending of the tibio-tarsal and metatarsal bones and is a common problem in meat-type poultry. It has a variety of possible causes (nutritional, rapid growth, management, etc.). Tibial dyschondroplasia causes backward bending or fracture of the top of the tibia. Slowing growth in young birds will help prevent leg deformity.

Other types of hock and stifle lameness and ruptured tendons are frequent in heavy roaster and turkeys and may be mainly due to injury as the result of heavy weight and fast growth, but some respond to added selenium or B vitamins.

Check for poor bone-breaking strength (osteoporosis) and, in young birds for rubbery bones, soft beaks, and beaded ribs which indicate calcium or Vit. D3 deficiency (rickets). Cage layer fatigue because of fragile bones may be due to phosphorus deficiency. Calcium and Vit. D3 deficiency also cause fragile bones (osteoporosis) in adults, but the most common cause is continuous high production.

Infectious stunting syndrome (malabsorption syndrome, fragile bones, osteoporosis) in young broilers is caused by intestinal damage from viral infection in young chicks. The chickens are small, poorly feathered and there is poorly digested food in the lower intestine. Osteomyelitis also causes fragile bones.

Curly-toe paralysis in young birds may be riboflavin deficiency, but in older birds and turkeys may be genetic or due to lack of roosts. Cracked feet and foot dermatitis may be pantothenic acid or biotin deficiency, but scaly leg is caused by mites.

Footpad dermatitis and hock lesion are often caused by poor litter conditions.

Toe injury in young birds may be cannibalism or mechanical injury. Arthritis in the feet or hocks or other joints suggests infectious synovitis (Mycoplasma synoviae) or E. coli or Staph. infection often with osteomyelitis.

Infection in the wing joints in pigeons is usually due to salmonella. In broilers, roaster and broiler breeders viral arthritis (reovirus infection) may cause lameness or ruptured tendons. Ruptured tendons are usually caused by rapid growth and large body size (heavy weight) and there is usually thickening of the tendon above the hock.

If growing birds are lame, and there is no evidence of infection or rickets, cut into the proximal tibia and look for necrosis caused by osteomyelitis or dyschondroplasia and split the spine at T4 to look for spondylolisthesis (kinky-back), a plug of cartilage impinging on the cord or consider Marek's disease.

Necrotic dermatitis is caused either by staph. or clostridium infection and is associated with immunosuppression (usually by CAV or IBD). Scabby-hip is usually from overcrowding, poor litter conditions, poor feathering or scratches. Dermatitis or granulation in the neck may be a vaccine reaction, or contaminated vaccine.

10. *Disturbances of the nervous system may cause incoordination, staggering, paralysis, walking backwards (with wings flapping for balance), tremors, stargazing, and other odd behaviour.*

    In case of lameness, paralysis, or incoordination, examine the sciatic nerves, spinal cord, and brain. Histologic examination will be required for diagnosis.

    ND may produce CNS disturbances in pigeons as well as nervous, respiratory, intestinal and reproductive lesions in chickens, pheasants, turkeys, and wild and cage birds of all ages.

    Range paralysis is a form of Marek's disease affecting the peripheral and central nervous system causing lameness, incoordination and paralysis. Marek's can also cause botulism-like paralysis and transient paralysis.

    Vitamin E deficiency (avian encephalomalacia) causes soft, dark areas of hemorrhage in the cerebellum which may be visible grossly. B vitamin deficiency (thiamine and other) may also cause nervous signs.

    Avian encephalomyelitis (AE) (epidemic tremor) affects birds up to 3-4 weeks old from non-immune parents.

    Arsenilic acid and other feed additives and toxins (botulism, lead) may cause CNS disturbances, while others like the ionophores and coffee weed seeds (Cassia) cause nerve or muscle damage. Bacterial infection (pasteurella, pseudomonas, salmonella, staph, etc.) and fungi (aspergillus, etc.) also cause meningoencephalitis, occasionally in outbreak proportions.

PARASITIC DISEASES (EXTERNAL)

Poultry Mites

All classes of poultry are susceptible to mites, some of which are blood-suckers, while others burrow into the skin or live on or in the feathers. Others occur in the air passages and in the lungs, liver and other internal organs. Poultry mites cause retarded growth, reduced egg production, lowered vitality, damaged plumage and even death. Much of the injury, consisting of constant irritation and loss of blood, is not apparent without careful examination. Of primary concern to the poultryman is the Northern Fowl Mite (Ornithonyssus sylviarum) which is a frequent and serious pest of chickens. Heavy infestations result in low condition of the birds and lower egg production, as well as a scabby skin condition.

The mite remains on the bird and does more damage than any other species of mite. The mite does not leave the host bird, as do may species of mites, and can be observed on birds in large numbers during daylight hours. It prefers the feathers below the vent and around the tail, but can be found on all parts of the body. The mite is extremely small and a microscope or magnifying glass may be needed to see it.

The female northern fowl mite lays eggs on feathers where the young mites complete their development without leaving the host. Since they remain on the fowl most of the time, treatment of the birds is necessary to destroy the mites. The Common Chicken Mite (Dermanyssus gallinae) is the most common mite found on all types of poultry. It is a blood-sucker, and when present in large numbers, loss of blood and irritation may be sufficient to cause anemia. Egg production is seriously reduced.

This mite feeds at night, and usually remains hidden in cracks and crevices during the day. It attacks birds at night while they are on the roost. In heavy infestations, some mites may remain on the birds during the day. About a day after feeding, the female lays eggs in cracks and crevices of the house. The eggs hatch and the mites develop into adults within about a week. During cold weather, the cycle is slower. A poultry house remains infested four to five months after birds are removed. Since the mite feeds on wild birds, these birds may be responsible for spreading infestations. However, it is more likely that spread of the mite is promoted by using contaminated coops. Human carriers are also important. Since these mites do not stay on the birds during the day, apply treatments to houses and equipment as well as the birds.

The Scaly-Leg Mite (Knemidocoptes mutans) lives under the scales on feet and legs of poultry. It also may attach to the comb and wattles. It causes a thickening of scales on the feet and legs that gives the impression that the scales are protruding directly outward, rather that laying flat on the limb. It spends its entire life cycle on the birds and spreads mainly by direct contact. The Depluming Mite (Knemidocoptes laevis, variety gallinae) causes severe irritation by burrowing into the skin near the bases of feathers and frequently causes feathers to be pulled out or broken.

The mite is barely visible to the naked eye and can be found in follicles at the base of the feathers. The mites crawl around the birds at times, spreading from bird to bird.

The most effective treatment for all mite species is a regular inspection and spraying programme of both the birds and their premises. An appropriate solution of permethrin, when sprayed on the birds, will eliminate all mites that infest the bird.

The spraying of all facilities will ensure that any mites hiding in cracks and crevices will be destroyed. The treatment should be repeated on a one to two month schedule or whenever populations of the mites are detected.

Mites

One of the most common problems encountered when raising and keeping poultry is mites. There are several kinds of mites that will infest your birds.

Where do they come from? They can be brought in via wild birds, such as starlings, sparrows, crows, swallows, etc. They can be picked up at poultry shows, sales, auctions, anywhere there is contact with other avian life. They can be carried in with rodents who enter the coops in search of food. Early intervention is necessary to prevent illness and debilitation in your flock.

How do you know what to look for? Chicken mites are the most common. They live on the skin of the birds, in the nest boxes, and in the bedding. They tend to be nocturnal, and will suck blood from the chicken while it sleeps. They are very small, and initially yellow/gray in colour, but will darken as they feed. Removing the chicken mite is most effectively directed at the coop than the birds themselves.

Poultry Lice

There are many different forms of lice that will infest poultry. Each region will have variations in which strain is the most predominate. What you will see that is common to all of them is that they are small wingless insects. They have chewing mouth parts, which differs from the sucking mouth parts of a mite. You can see a louse as it moves on the skin by parting the feathers, especially at the head, under the wings, and around the vent. Lice do not suck blood. They feed on dry skin scales and feathers. They cause irritation by the act of movement on the skin of the bird, and the action of the mouth. This, while not as direct a loss to the bird, will cause appetite loss and the resulting weakness, lowered egg production, and susceptibility to illness.

Treatment

Treatment for all of the above pests must be undertaken to prevent loss to the flock. There are many products on the market that have been effective for this. Products such as Sevin dust have been used effectively on both coops and directly on the birds. This is a Carbaryl based insecticide that will directly kill the existing mites. Re-treatment is usually necessary due to the eggs that will hatch and reinfest the birds and coop. Orange Guard is effective organic non-toxic treatment for the coop itself, but cannot be used directly on the birds. All will respond to pour-on medications, such as Eprinex.

Scaly leg mites can be treated with a direct contact treatment. Petrolatum jelly, vegetable, mineral, linseed oil are effective when directly applied to the legs and repeated every two days till scales are smooth again. Adding 1 part kerosene to two parts oil has been noted to be effective as well.

Prevention

Prevention of mite and louse infestation is difficult. Early detection remains the best way to control these pests. Keeping the coops and bedding clean and fresh, periodic scrubbing of the coop and nesting boxes with soap and water, and regular inspecting of your flock to catch the problem before harm is done to the chickens.

Poultry Lice

The primary effects of lice on their hosts are the irritations they cause. The birds become restless and do not feed or sleep well. They may injure themselves or damage their feathers by pecking or scratching areas irritated by lice. Body weight and egg production may drop. All lice infecting poultry and birds are the chewing type. Mites may be confused with lice, but mites suck blood. In general, each species of lice is confined to a particular kind of poultry, although some may pass from one kind to another when birds are different species; turkeys have three common species.

All species of poultry lice have certain common habits. All live continuously on feathered hosts and soon die if removed. The eggs are attached to the feathers. Young lice resemble adults except in colour and size. Lice differ in preferred locations on the host, and these preferences have given rise to the common names applied to various species. In general, the incubation period of lice eggs is four to seven days, and development of the lice between hatching and the adult stage requires about twenty-one days. Mating takes place on the fowl, and egg laying begins two to three days after lice mature. The number of eggs probably ranges from fifty to three-hundred per female louse.

As the name suggests, the Head Louse (Cuclotogaster heterographa) is found mainly on the head, although it occurs occasionally on the neck and elsewhere. It usually is located near the skin in the down or at the base of the feathers on the top and back of the head and beneath the beak. In fact, the head of the louse often is found so close to the skin that poultrymen may think it is attached to the skin or is sucking blood. Although it does not suck blood, the head louse is very irritating and ranks first among lice as a pest of young chickens and turkeys. Heavily infested chicks soon become droopy and weak and may die before they are a month old. When the chickens become fairly well feathered, head lice decrease but may increase again when the fowls reach maturity.

This louse is oblong, grayish and about 1/10-inch long. The pearly-white eggs are attached singly to the down or at the base of the small feathers on the head. They hatch within five days into minute, pale, translucent lice resembling adults in shape. The Body Louse (Menacanthus stramineus) of chickens prefers to stay on the skin rather than on the feathers. It chooses parts of the body that are not densely feathered, such as the area below the vent. In heavy infestations, it may be found on the breast, under the wings and on other parts of the body, including the head.

When the feathers are parted, straw-coloured body lice may be seen running rapidly on the skin in search of cover. Eggs are deposited in clusters near the base of small feathers, particularly below the vent, or in young fowls, frequently on the head or throat. Eggs hatch in about a week and lice reach maturity within twenty days. This is the most common louse infesting grown chickens. When present in large numbers, the skin is irritated greatly and scabs may result, especially below the vent.

The Shaft Louse or small body louse (Menopon gallinae) is similar in appearance to the body louse, but smaller. It has a habit of resting on the body feather shafts of chickens where it may be seen running rapidly towards the body when feathers are parted suddenly. Sometimes as many as a dozen lice may be seen scurrying down a feather shaft. Since the shaft louse apparently feeds on parts of the feathers, it is found in limited numbers on turkeys, guinea fowl and ducks kept in close association with chickens. It does not infest young birds until they become well feathered.

The same control measures used to eliminate mite populations is effective for treating lice. It is more important to apply the insecticides directly to the bird's body rather than the premises.

Poultry lice spend their entire lives on the body of the chicken. They cannot survive without remaining on the host. When looking for them, they prefer hanging out near the vent, but can be found under the wings and on the head as well. Sometime, you will discover the eggs first. Where the skin meets the feathers, you will see tiny clumped little white eggs at the base. Poultry lice can be seen walking around on the skin of the chicken as they feast on dead skin, feathers and scabs. They will not suck blood but do ingest blood from irritated raw areas of the skin. This behaviour is very irritating to affected chickens and in severe cases be fatal. Chickens that have poultry lice can show an assortment of symptoms that are similar to a mite infestation and include:

- Weight loss
- Decreased appetite
- Drop in egg production
- Feather loss around areas of infestation
- Feathers that have an appearance as though they have been eaten by a moth
- Irritated inflamed raw skin initially near the vent.

Prevention

1. *Sanitation.* Keep the coop and run clean and prevent overcrowding in your flock. Here is how we clean our coop.
2. *Inspections.* Inspect your chickens at least every 1-2 weeks for the presence of lice or mites.
3. *Take preventative measures.* Add food grade diatomaceous earth to your coop and nesting box bedding. Add it to the dust bathing areas too.
4. *Quarantine* and inspect any new birds that you are adding to your flock for at least 2 weeks. Treat them if necessary.
5. Prevent wild birds from nesting in or near your coop and run.

Treatment

1. *Clean.* Thoroughly clean your entire coop and run and add food grade diatomaceous earth (DE) to all the bedding.
2. *Treat.* Dust each flock member with DE or a garden dust such as Sevin-5 per cent. I have no personal experiences with Sevin but many on backyardchickens.com swear by it. Older labels deemed it safe for pets there are alternatives, I would try other methods prior to using Sevin dust. Permethrin is also available as well as Manna Pro's Poultry Protector. Cover your mouth and nose to avoid inhaling the dust products and also avoid the head of your chicken. I prefer the DE and Poultry Protector as they are safe to use around the flock's food and water.
3. *Re-treat.* The life cycle of poultry lice is two weeks. Mark your calendar and repeat steps 1 and 2 to ensure that you have eradicated the lice.
4. *Prevention.*

DISEASES FROM MISCELLANEOUS CAUSES

Cage Layer Fatigue

Rickets and cage layer fatigue are nutritional diseases seen in chickens, turkeys and ducks that results in soft bones, with the leg bones often becoming bowed and hampering the bird's ability to stand and walk. The term rickets is generally used to describe the condition in young poultry, while osteomalacia is often the term used for the disease in adult birds. Caged layer fatigue is a related condition observed in caged laying hens, usually around peak egg production, that may also be associated with osteoporosis, a condition causing brittle bones as a result of reduced bone density.

What causes rickets and cage layer fatigue? Rickets is caused by a deficiency or imbalance of circulating calcium, vitamin D3 or phosphorous. It can be caused by an imbalanced or deficient diet, some medications and also some mould toxins. Caged layer fatigue is thought to be caused primarily by depletion of body stores of calcium as a result of delay in feeding high calcium feeds during high egg production or a metabolic malfunction that impairs calcium absorption or bone calcification during this production stage.

Prevention and Treatment of Rickets and Cage Layer Fatigue

For normal bone calcification, calcium and phosphorous need to be supplied not only in adequate amounts but in a ratio to each other of about 2:1. Excess of either calcium or phosphorous can cause rickets. Vitamin D3 plays a critical role in regulating the absorption and metabolism of calcium. Therefore, in addition to ensuring that poultry diets have an appropriate level and balance of calcium and phosphorous, they must be adequate in vitamin D3. Bone mineralisation is a constant process and so correction of dietary deficiencies or imbalances can ease the condition if caught early enough. Mould or fungal toxins, called mycotoxins, can have a range of effects on poultry including interfering with the absorption of nutrients. Rickets caused through the presence of dietary mycotoxins can be treated by replacing the toxin-contaminated feed and by supplementing vitamin D3 to three or fourfold of the usual levels. There is a higher incidence of bone calcification problems in high producing layer hens housed in cages rather than floor-based housing systems, hence the term cage layer fatigue. This indicated the role of exercise in preventing or treating this condition.

Cannibalism

Cannibalism is a problem that is associated with large poultry flocks where the birds kept in close confinement peck at associated birds. This can result in significant mortality within the flock when a wound is generated and it will also cause a decrease in egg production as the hen pecked birds become stressed. This is a vice which is usually precipitated by some aspect of management or environment which the birds are subjected to. Under the intensive management conditions used by today's industry this condition can occur in all ages of birds and in many species. It has been determined, however that the light breeds, such as the leghorns that are used in table egg production, are more susceptible than the heavier breeds. These lighter breeds are characterized by their flighty nature and are hypersensitive to environmental factors.

The behavioural problem of cannibalism in the poultry industry can include the following vices:

- Toe picking in chicks
- Feather pulling in older birds from the head, tail or body
- Vent picking in older birds.

Feather pulling and vent pecking may be difficult and time consuming behaviours to observe in a flock, but the cannibalism can be clearly recognized when culled birds or moralities in the flock have had much of the intestine removed through the vent. Cannibalism can also take a number of forms among the birds in a flock and can be presented in the following ways:

- A dominant bird pecking at a more submissive member of the flock
- Mutual pecking where birds in close proximity peck at each other
- On rare occasions young chicks may peck their own toes.

The causes of this vice are not well understood, but the onset of cannibalism has been attributed to a number of things which are outlined below:

- The problem may simply arise because of the normal pecking behaviour of this type ofanimal when searching for food or exploring an environment. The birds are kept in barren, crowded conditions and may have little else to peck besides their pen mates. Once one hen has picked up this technique other hens, observing the behaviour, will learn from the initial pecker and a serious episode will develop.
- A lack or a deficiency of nutrients in a poultry ration may result in the birds becoming irritated which can subsequently lead

to cannibalism in the flock. Usually when diet formulation is involved in the outbreak the imbalance is in the protein or the sodium level of the ration. Deficiencies can also be caused by insufficient feeding and water space.

- An abrupt change in the palatability or form of a flock's ration may also be a contributing factor in the onset of cannibalism as the birds might impulsively seek alternative sources of food.
- Poor ventilation, high temperature, low humidity, excessive population density, and excess illumination are all factors in the flock's environment that may precipitate an outbreak of this vice, especially with the lighter breeds.
- During egg laying the cloaca may become damaged and distended especially with the passage of large eggs and this protrusion of the vent may be an attractant to other birds due to its stark colour difference against the white body.

The onset of this vice can be prevented by paying particular attention to the dietary factors (protein, sodium, and palatability), the environmental factors (ventilation, temperature, humidity, population density, and lighting) and the feeding and water space that is available for each bird. With highly intensive operations the light intensity should be reduced, perhaps by changing to a light which is of a red hue.

The most common and cost effective mode of prevention is the use of beak trimming. Beak trimming is usually done at 4-6 weeks of age and the procedure requires that two thirds of the upper mandible be removed. Beak trimming is usually done with an electric debeaking machine which is available commercially. This procedure will not eliminate the abnormal behaviour entirely but the birds are less able to inflict damage. A controversial approach is the use aluminum rings which are fixed to the upper beaks of the birds, but this has already been banned in some countries.

If an outbreak of cannibalism has already been initiated in a flock a manager may want to try to increase the searching aspect of feeding. Other control methods include increasing feed availability, reducing group size, adding litter, and providing distractants such as straw bales. Some managers of turkey flocks also will use a tar-like spray which deters cannibalism due to its offensive odour and taste. It should be remembered when approaching a problem of cannibalism in the poultry industry that the best method of control is to prevent it from starting at all, since once it has begun it will be very difficult to stop.

Causes of Cannibalism

Cannibalism is caused by a combination of genetic and environmental factors. Although the exact etiology is unknown, many management conditions and genetics can predispose a flock to an outbreak.

Prevention

Outbreaks can occur in the best-managed flock. However, problems are less likely to arise if preventative measures are in place. The first step in a cannibalism control programme is to select a genetic stock that is not prone to cannibalism and then give the birds the best care possible, including adequate feed, carefully managed lighting, safe housing and environmental enrichment.

Providing a complete ration to meet the nutrient needs for age and type of flock is also very important. Cannibalism has been linked to deficiencies in protein, sodium and phosphorus. Protein requirements change as chicks grow and should be adjusted based on a recommended feeding schedule. Adequate feeder space for all birds to eat simultaneously helps prevent underweight birds that are frequently victims of cannibalism.

Both lighting schedules and light intensity can influence cannibalistic behaviour. Photostimulation programmes should be delayed until birds are physically mature, after 20 weeks of age. Dim lights are often used in combination with beak trimming to prevent cannibalism, but lighting should be bright enough to permit daily inspection of flocks and facilities. If reduced lighting is used, 5-10 lux (about 0.5 to 1.0 foot candles) from incandescent or fluorescent bulbs is recommended (example: just barely enough to read a newspaper). Cannibalism is a learned behaviour and, once established, can spread throughout a flock.

Because chickens are attracted to blood, outbreaks can be initiated by the injury of one bird and subsequent pecking of the injury by a flock or cage mate. That means it is important to keep bird enclosures in good repair to prevent injury. Loose wires on cages or pens can puncture the skin and cause bleeding. A bird that gets snagged or caught can tear its skin or lose feathers as it attempts to escape.

Older cages and enclosures should be replaced before injuries and pecking become common. Cannibalistic chickens, injured birds, victims of cannibalism and dead birds should be quickly removed from the flock. Environmental enrichment is the practice of putting objects in the cage or pen to provide interest and a greater variety of behavioural outlets. For hens, environmental enrichments that reduce the incidence of cannibalism include nest boxes, perches, foraging opportunities and other things that might redirect pecking away from flock mates.

A dark nest box provides a safe place for egg laying and prevents exposure of the everted cloaca during oviposition to potentially cannibalistic flock mates. Because the cloaca is highly attractive for pecking, some outbreaks of cannibalism begin during oviposition. Hens can escape aggressive vent pecking by perching high enough off of the ground that they cannot be reached by hens on the floor. Pullets are more likely to use perches as a refuge if they are reared with them from an early age.

Pullets reared on a litter type that is attractive for scratching and pecking are less likely to develop cannibalistic behaviour. A chicken's natural behaviour includes spending a considerable portion of the day searching for food. When the environment is not suitable for the expression of normal foraging behaviour, pecking can sometimes be redirected towards flock mates and this may lead to cannibalism. It is important to provide foraging opportunities such as straw, green leafy vegetables or grass clippings, or to feed small grains in deep litter. A mash diet, rather than pelleted feed, may also help prevent outbreaks of cannibalism because chickens sift through the variety of ground particles and take longer to consume their feed.

Enrichment devices made of string have also been shown to redirect pecking. Four to eight lengths of white polypropylene twine hung in the cage or pen should elicit pecking and may help prevent aggressive pecking towards flock mates. Enrichment devices that are moved or changed periodically are more effective in keeping the birds' attention. Ideally, poultry should be allowed protected outdoor access where they can display the full range of their natural foraging and exploratory behaviours.

A combination of careful selection of genetic stock and good management practices prevents most cannibalism; however, beak trimming is often practiced as a preventative method. The practice of beak trimming is associated with both acute and chronic pain and should not be practiced indiscriminately. Neuromas, tangles of severed nerve endings in the amputated beak stump, sometimes result from beak trimming.

Until alternatives to beak trimming are developed, the potential painfulness of this practice should be weighed against the likelihood of a cannibalism outbreak when making the decision to beak trim. Current research aimed at preventing cannibalism through genetic selection of more docile stock may prevent the need to beak trim in the future.

Control of a Cannibalism Outbreak

Although it is better to prevent cannibalism, if an outbreak does occur, it is essential to stop the behaviour quickly before it spreads throughout the flock. A variety of methods are available to help accomplish this objective, although it is difficult to stop a substantial outbreak altogether. Some corrective steps include:

- Separate birds doing the severe feather pecking, especially if directed at the injuries or vents of other birds.

- Add enrichments, especially foraging-related devices.
- Add additional feed and water space.
- Add nest boxes and perches.
- Use an antibiotic wound spray on the everted cloaca of hens with vent trauma (in small flock situations).
- Consider therapeutic beak trimming.

Beak Trimming

The avian beak is highly innervated and, like the human hand, is very sensitive to touch, temperature and pressure. Chickens use their beaks not only for gathering food but also for exploring and manipulating objects in the environment, pre-ening, dustbathing, nesting and social interactions. Beak trimming is not only painful, it deprives the bird of important sensory information. However, if alternatives have been exhausted, a careful beak trimming programme will prevent most cannibalism outbreaks.

Cannibalism does not spread as efficiently in caged systems for laying hens, given sufficient access to feed and water space and low numbers of birds per cage. Medium hybrid laying hen stock should not need beak trimming when housed in battery cage systems. However, White Leghorn light hybrids housed at high cage stocking densities (less than 70 square inches per hen) can experience very high mortality from cannibalism.

Although stocking densities greater than 86 in2/hen are not recommended, crowding above this level without extensive measures to prevent cannibalism necessitates beak trimming. If the decision is to beak trim, the procedure should be done between seven and 10 days of age and only by properly trained personnel.

Beak trimming errors can result in additional pain and suffering to an already stressful procedure or may fail to prevent cannibalism. It is important to remove the correct amount of beak. Severe beak trims result in neuroma formation and the build up of scar tissue; but a conservative trim of only one- fourth to one-third of the upper beak (measured from the tip to the nostril) and slightly less of the lower beak usually prevents this outcome. The beak should be trimmed at an angle from top to bottom to remove less of the lower mandible. A heated blade is usually used to trim beaks. However, new technologies using lasers and infrared beams are currently being researched, and producers should be prepared to adopt these new methods if they become available. Bleeding will occur if the blade on a hot blade trimmer is too hot or too cold or if environmental temperatures cause the flock to become overheated.

Fatty Liver Hemorrhagic Syndrome

This problem is commonly referred to as Fatty Liver Hemorrhagic Syndrome. It results when large amounts of fat is deposited in the hen's liver and abdomen. The liver becomes soft and easily damaged and is more prone to bleeding. The liver contains many blood vessels that rupture easily during egg laying, resulting in massive bleeding and death. When laying hens are fed diets containing high levels of dietary energy the hens tend to deposit excess energy as fat deposits in their bodies, especially the liver. The problem is more common when feeds containing high levels of corn or other high energy ingredients is fed. Therefore, it is not advisable to feed chopped corn as the sole feedstuff to laying hens.

The condition is most often seen in birds that appear to be healthy and in a state of high egg production. Non-laying hens will not eat as much of the high-energy feed and therefore are not affected as much as high producing hens. The problem can be prevented by feeding complete layer diets that contain the proper amounts of all nutrients. Corn is an excellent ingredient for poultry diets, but should not be fed as the only feed for hens. Therefore, do not feed corn as the only feed or in combination with complete feeds.

Causes

Excessive dietary energy intake is believed to be the cause of fatty liver hemorrhagic syndrome. Heredity may also play a role, but it is not the entire cause for the disease. Birds housed in cages will more likely be affected because they are unable to exercise to burn off the extra dietary energy. Walking hens are less likely to develop this problem. The disease is observed most often in birds that appear to be healthy and in a state of high egg production. As a result, death can occur quite unexpectedly.

Symptoms

Affected birds are usually overweight and may also have pale combs. Generally, however, the disease has few or no symptoms prior to the bird's death.

Treatment

The use of L-Tryptophan in the diet can decrease the syndrome.

□

2

Viral Diseases in Poultry

This Action focused on Infectious Bursal Diseases (IBDV) and Chicken Anaemia (CAV), two important viral diseases in poultry production. An evaluation of the economic impact of these viral diseases on the poultry industry in the participating countries was performed but complicated by the multifaceted nature of the infection and by lack of tools, for example, serology can not differentiate between infected and healthy (vaccinated) flocks.

Recommendations and guidelines concerning vaccines were developed for the European Agency for the Evaluation of Medicinal Products (EMEA) in London. These recommendations were key factors in the recent update and changes of the monographs of IBDV and CAV.

The scientists participating in this Action produced a handbook with state- of-the-art knowledge and recommen-dations for future research and current practices, providing guidelines for the Office International de Epizooties-Paris (OIE) and the EU.

The network resulted in standardisation of tools and nomenclature. One of the results is an annual ring trial for serological tests with 96 laboratories participating. In addition, one ring test on bursal lesions scoring was completed in all the participating countries in the Action. Attention was paid to the transfer of knowledge and technology, especially to the poultry industry. A total 14 companies participated in this Action.

AVIAN POX

Avian pox is a relatively slow-spreading viral disease in birds, characterized by wart-like nodules on the skin and diphtheritic necrotic membranes lining the mouth and upper respiratory system. It has been present in birds since the earliest history. Mortality is not usually significant unless the respiratory involvement is marked. The disease may occur in any age of bird, at any time. Avian pox is caused by a virus of which there are at least three different strains or types; fowl pox virus, pigeon pox virus and canary pox virus. Although some workers include turkey pox virus as a distinct strain, many feel that is identical to fowl pox virus.

Each virus strain is infective for a number of species of birds. Natural occurring pox in chickens, turkeys and other domestic fowl is considered to be caused by fowl pox virus. Fowl pox can be transmitted by direct or indirect contact. The virus is highly resistant in dried scabs and under certain conditions may survive for months on contaminated premises. The disease may be transmitted by a number of species of mosquitoes. Mosquitoes can harbor infective virus for a month or more after feeding on affected birds. After the infection is introduced, it spreads within the flock by mosquitoes as well as direct and indirect contact. Recovered birds do not remain carriers.

Since fowl pox usually spreads slowly, a flock may be affected for several months. The course of the disease in the individual bird takes three to five weeks. Affected young birds are retarded in growth. Laying birds experience a drop in egg production. Birds of all ages that have oral or respiratory system involvement have difficulty eating and breathing. The disease manifests itself in one or two ways, cutaneous pox (dry form) or diphtheritic pox (wet form). Dry pox starts as small whitish foci that develop into wart-like nodules. The nodules eventually are sloughed and scab formation precedes final healing. Lesions are most commonly seen on the featherless parts of the body (comb, wattles, ear lobes, eyes, and sometimes the feet).

Wet pox is associated with the oral cavity and the upper respiratory tract, particularly the larynx and trachea. The lesions are diphtheritic in character and involve the mucous membranes to such a degree that when removed, an ulcerated or eroded area is left. Fowl pox is readily diagnosed on the basis of flock history and presence of typical lesions. In some cases, laboratory diagnosis by tissue or transmission studies is necessary.

There is no treatment for fowl pox. Disease control is accomplished best by preventative vaccination since ordinary management and sanitation practices will not prevent it. Several kinds of vaccines are available and are effective if used properly. Vaccination of broilers is not usually required unless the mosquito population is high or infections have occurred previously. The chicks may be vaccinated as young as one day of age by using the wing-web method and using a one needle applicator. All replacement chickens are vaccinated against fowl pox when the birds are six to ten weeks of age. One application of fowl pox vaccine results in permanent immunity.

NEWCASTLE DISEASE

Newcastle disease is a contagious viral infection causing a respiratory nervous disorder in several species of fowl including chickens and turkeys.

Different types or strains of the virus (varying in their ability to cause nervous disorder, visceral lesions and death) have been recognized. The most severe strain is called viscerotropic velogenic Newcastle disease (VVND) and is kept from birds in the U.S. by enforcement of strict quarantines at our national borders. It is often referred to as 'Exotic Newcastle Disease' and infection of susceptible fowl with this form usually causes high mortality.

A milder form of the disease is called 'mesogenic' Newcastle disease and is the most serious strain found in the U.S. Newcastle disease is highly contagious. All birds in a flock usually become infected within three to four days. The virus can be transmitted by contaminated equipment, shoes, clothing and free-flying birds. During the active respiratory stage, it can be transmitted through the air. The virus is not thought to travel any great distance by this method. Recovered birds are not considered carriers and the virus usually does not live longer than thirty days on the premises.

Signs of Newcastle disease are not greatly different from those of other respiratory diseases. The signs most frequently observed are nasal discharge, excessive mucous in the trachea, cloudy air sacs, casts or plugs in the air passages of the lungs and cloudiness in the cornea of the eye. The disease in young chickens begins with difficult breathing, gasping and sneezing. This phase continues for ten to fourteen days and may be followed by nervous symptoms. If nervous disorders develop, they may consist of paralysis of one or both wings and legs or a twisting of the head and neck. The head often is drawn over the back or down between the legs. Mortality may vary from none to total loss of the flock.

In adult chickens, respiratory symptoms predominate. Only rarely do nervous disorders develop. If the flock is laying, egg production usually drops rapidly. When this occurs, it takes four weeks or longer for the flock to return to the former production rate. During the outbreak, small, soft-shelled, off- coloured and irregular-shaped eggs are produced. Mortality in adult birds is usually low but may be fairly high from some virus strains. In turkeys, the symptoms are usually mild and may be unnoticed unless nervous disorders develop. During an outbreak, turkeys will produce eggs with a chalky white shell. Reduced production in breeder flocks is the main economic loss from this disease in turkeys.

The flock history, signs of a respiratory nervous disorder and other typical lesions often may be sufficient to allow a tentative diagnosis. Usually, however, the disease cannot be differentiated from infectious bronchitis and some of the other respiratory infections, except by laboratory methods. Vaccination is practiced widely and is the recommended method for prevention. Several types of vaccines are available but the most successful and widely used is the mild live virus vaccine known as the B1 and La Sota types. The vaccines may be used by drops into the nostril or eye, addition to the drinking water or applied in spray form. Broiler chickens are usually vaccinated when seven to ten days of age. Chickens kept for egg production are usually vaccinated at least three times. The vaccine is given when birds are approximately seven days, again at about four weeks and a third time at about four months of age. Revaccination while in lay is commonly practiced. Vaccination is not widely used in turkeys. It is used to protect egg producing breeder flocks. One dose of the mild type vaccine is given after selecting breeder birds.

There is no treatment for Newcastle disease. The disease does not always respect even the best management programmes, but good 'biosecurity' practices will help reduce the possibility of exposure to Newcastle disease virus.

INFECTIOUS BRONCHITIS

Infectious bronchitis is an extremely contagious respiratory disease of chickens characterized by coughing, sneezing and rales (rattling). It is caused by a virus that affects chickens only. Other fowl or laboratory animals cannot be infected with this virus. Several distinct strains of the virus exist.

Infectious bronchitis is considered the most contagious of poultry diseases. When it occurs, all susceptible birds on the premises become infected, regardless of sanitary or quarantine precautions. The disease can spread through the air and can 'jump' considerable distances during an active outbreak. It can also be spread by mechanical means such as on clothing, poultry crates and equipment. The disease is not egg transmitted and the virus will survive for probably no more than one week in the house when poultry are not present. It is easily destroyed by heat and ordinary disinfectants. The infection is confined to the respiratory system. Symptoms are difficult breathing, gasping, sneezing and rales. Some birds may have a slight watery nasal discharge. The disease never causes nervous symptoms. It prevails for ten to fourteen days in a flock and symptoms lasting longer than this are from some other cause.

In chickens under three weeks of age, mortality may be as high as thirty or forty per cent. The disease does not cause a significant mortality in birds over five weeks of age. Feed consumption decreases sharply and growth is retarded. When infectious bronchitis occurs in a laying flock, production usually drops to near zero with a few days. Four weeks or more may be required before the flock returns to production. Some flocks never regain an economical rate of lay. During an outbreak, small, soft-shelled, irregular- shaped eggs are produced.

Infectious bronchitis is difficult to differentiate from many of the other respiratory diseases. For this reason, a definite diagnosis usually requires a laboratory analysis. Infectious bronchitis is highly contagious and does not always respect sanitary barriers. Vaccinate chickens being retained as layers.

Whether broilers should be vaccinated depends upon many factors and is an individual decision. Numerous vaccines are available commercially. Most of them represent a modified or selected strain of the infectious bronchitis virus. The vaccine used should contain virus known to be present in the area. All vaccines contain live virus and those that give the best protection are also capable of producing symptoms and reducing egg production. The vaccine virus will spread to other susceptible birds. Vaccine is usually added to the drinking water, but may be dropped into the eye or nostril or used as a spray.

There is no treatment for this disease. In young chickens it is helpful to increase the brooder temperature and provide as nearly ideal environmental conditions as possible.

QUAIL BRONCHITIS

Quail bronchitis is a contagious, highly fatal disease in young bobwhite quail. The virus causing this disease also infects chickens and turkey. This agent is also known as a CELO (Chick Embryo Lethal Organism) virus. It has been isolated from chicken eggs but does not produce a recognizable disease in chickens or turkeys. This agent may play a part in respiratory diseases and in infertility problems, but its importance must be established by additional research. It is important because it is one of the agents that may be isolated from birds with respiratory symptoms and is difficult to separate from other agents such as infectious bronchitis virus.

LYMPHOID LEUKOSIS

Characteristically, lymphoid leukosis is a disease of adult chickens; however, the disease appears to be increasing in importance for turkeys and game birds. Although the virus of lymphoid leukosis can produce various responses (blood, bone, lymph), the lymphoid tumour response is the most common. The disease is transmitted in a variety of ways. The causative viral agent is passed out of the body of infected birds via eggs and feces. The virus may be transmitted mechanically from infected birds to susceptibles by blood- sucking parasites or by man in such procedures as fowl pox vaccination.

Lymphoid leukosis characteristically produces lymphoid tumors, particularly in the liver and spleen. The tumors may also affect other visceral organs such as ovary and lungs. Affected birds may die without preliminary symptoms, but the disease usually is chronic in nature and affected birds show loss of appetite, progressive emaciation and diarrhea. Clinically affected birds invariably die. Losses due to the disease are most severe shortly after onset of egg production, but losses will continue for as long as the flock is retained. Total loss may approach twenty per cent during the life of a flock. Clinical diagnosis of lymphoid leukosis is based upon flock history and disease manifestations. The lymphoid disease cannot be readily distinguished from the visceral response to Marek's disease; however, there are some features that aid in differential diagnosis. There is no treatment for lymphoid leukosis. Although the disease cannot be prevented completely, there are certain steps that can be taken to help control the level of infection within a flock. Some steps are:

- Buy resistant strains of birds since genetic resistance is a deterrent,
- Brood in isolation and do not mix birds of different ages, especially through six weeks of age,
- Keep the incubator clean and disinfected,
- Control blood-sucking parasites,
- Good care, limiting stress, and adequate ration will be of benefit.

MAREK'S DISEASE (VISCERAL LEUKOSIS)

Marek's disease is characteristically a disease of young chickens but older birds can also be affected. In contrast to the lymphoid leukosis tumour response, Marek's disease may be observed in more diverse locations. Marek's disease is caused by a virus belonging to the Herpes virus group. Much is known about the transmission of the virus; however, it appears that the virus is concentrated in the feather follicles and shed in the dander (sloughed skin and feather cells). The virus has a long survival time in dander since viable virus can be isolated from houses that have been depopulated for many months.

The usual mode of transmission is by aerosols containing infected dander and dust. Young birds are most susceptible to infection by Marek's disease; however, since the incubation period is short, clinical symptoms can appear much earlier than in the case with lymphoid leukosis. Marek's disease may produce a variety of clinical responses, all lymphoid in character. These are acute visceral, neural, ocular, skin or combinations of the responses that can be seen.

Marek's of the visceral type is characterized by widespread involvement with lesions commonly seen in gonads, liver, spleen, kidney and occasionally heart, lungs and muscles. The disease is often acute, with apparently healthy birds dying very rapidly with massive internal tumors. The disease may appear in broiler-age birds but the most severe losses occur in replacement pullet flocks prior to onset of egg production.

The neural type of Marek's is typified by progressive paralysis of the wings, legs and neck. Loss of body weight, anemia, laboured respiration and diarrhea are common symptom. If lesions are present, they are confined to the nerve trunks and plexes enervating the paralyzed extremities. Frequently no gross lesions can be observed. Ocular (eye) leukosis or 'gray-eye' is usually seen in early maturity. Morbidity and mortality are usually low but may approach twenty-five per cent in some flocks. It is characterized by the spotty depigmentation or diffuse graying of the iris in the eye. The pupil develops an irregular shape and fails to react to light. Emaciation diarrhea and death follow.

Skin leukosis produces the most severe losses in broilers. The losses result from high condemnations at the processing plant. Enlargement of the feather follicles due to accumulations of lymphocytes is the typical lesion. This is the most infective virus since it is produced in the regions of the feather follicles and is shed with the skin dander. Acute Marek's disease can be extremely rapid in its course, producing mortality in apparently healthy birds. However, in some cases the lesions may regress and clinically affected birds may make complete recoveries.

Diagnosis is based upon flock history and disease manifestations. Accurate diagnosis may depend on results of laboratory procedures. As is the case with lymphoid leukosis, there is no treatment for Marek's disease. A vaccine is available that is extremely effective (90 per cent +) in the prevention of Marek's disease. It is administered to day-old chickens as a subcutaneous injection while the birds are in the hatchery. Use of the vaccine requires strict accordance with manufacturer's recommendations in a sterile environment.

INFECTIOUS BURSAL DISEASE (GUMBORO)

Infectious bursal disease is an acute, highly contagious viral disease of young chickens. It is most often found in highly concentrated poultry producing areas. It causes marked morbidity and mortality in affected flocks. Although the disease causes severe losses, its affect on reducing the bird's ability to develop immunity to other diseases may be the most serious effect produced by this disease. The transmission or spread of the disease can occur by direct contact (bird to bird), contaminated litter and feces, caretaker, contaminated air, equipment, feed, servicemen and possible insects and wild birds. It is extremely contagious.

Birds have ruffled feathers, a slight tremor at onset of the disease, strained defecation, loss of appetite and are dehydrated. Affected birds have a tendency to sit and when forced to move, have an unsteady gait. Vent picking is common and a whitish diarrhea frequently develops. A sudden rise in body temperature is followed by a drop to subnormal temperature, prostration and death. Birds surviving the initial infection will recover rapidly within two weeks.

Postmortem lesions include dehydration and changes in the bursa, skeletal muscle, liver and kidneys. All affected birds have bursal changes characterized by swelling, change in shape (oblong), colour (pink, yellow, red, black) and the formation of a gelatinous film around the bursa. Within a few days the bursa shrinks to half its normal size or smaller. Diagnosis of infectious bursal disease is based on flock history and postmortem lesions. Laboratory procedures may be used to substantiate the diagnosis.

Vaccines are available but must be carefully used. If given correctly, good immunity can be developed. There is no specific treatment for infectious bursal disease and indiscriminate medication with certain drugs may severely aggravate mortality. Supportive measures such as increasing heat, ventilation and water consumption are beneficial.

NEWCASTLE DISEASE (NCD)

This disease spreads rapidly via airborne droplets spread by the coughing or sneezing of infected birds. The virus can be carried by wild birds, through contaminated eggs, and on clothing. As mortality is often 100 per cent in young chickens, NCD is probably the most important constraint to family poultry development. Birds of any age can be affected, although young ones are more susceptible. Mortality in older chickens is usually lower, but egg production is usually severely reduced.

The incubation period of three to five days is followed by dullness, coughing, sneezing and gasping. Rapid breathing is accompanied by a gurgling noise in the throat. The respiratory signs usually develop first and are sometimes followed by nervous signs, characterized by twisting of the neck, sometimes combined with dragging of wings and legs. Depending on the environment and the degree of resistance of the birds, not all symptoms may be shown, or they may be in a mild or subclinical form.

The twisting of the neck occurs only in birds that survive. Early loss of appetite results in a greenish diarrhoea. The most obvious diagnostic sign of NCD is very sudden, very high mortality, often with few symptoms having had time to develop.

Diagnosis of NCD can be difficult from just the symptoms, as they are so varied, and as many other diseases share the same symptoms.

The high incidence of ND among family free-range flocks is due to the following factors:

- The prevalence of virulent strains
- Continuous contact with other domestic and wild species of birds (such as ducks and pigeons) which can carry the virus without showing the disease
- Uncontrolled movement of birds between villages.

There is a seasonal pattern to outbreaks of NCD, influenced by:

- The arrival of migratory birds;
- Changes in climatic conditions leading to stress, which predisposes birds to the disease;
- Hot, dry and windy periods, which encourage airborne spread of the virus; and
- Overuse of the few supply points of water available (during the virus.

FOWL POX

Fowl pox is still prevalent in many poultry flocks for the following reasons: The fowl pox virus can remain alive in the pox scabs (which have fallen off the birds) for up to ten years, which contaminate the environment. Mosquitoes and other blood-sucking insects can transmit the virus. The disease tends to be seasonal, occurring after mosquito breeding times.

MYCOPLASMAL DISEASES

Mycoplasmas are not classified as bacteria or viruses, but as Pleuro-pneumonia-cocci-like organisms (PPLO). These are primarily associated with Chronic Respiratory Disease (CRD), a complex syndrome caused by Mycoplasma gallisepticum in partnership with bacteria (often E. coli), fungi and viruses (often Infectious Bronchitis). M. gallisepticum can be transmitted through the egg. Multi-age flocks, nutritional deficiency and water deprivation are important factors in the epidemiology of the disease in rural poultry flocks.

DUCK VIRAL HEPATITIS

A viral disease of ducks occurring worldwide and previously a scheduled disease in UK. Morbidity is around 100 per cent and mortality 0-95 per cent. The disease is transmitted by infected ducks and other waterfowl and spreads rapidly, recovered birds carrying the virus for 8 weeks. The infective agent, a picornavirus may also survive for ten weeks in brooders and five weeks in faeces. A different picornavirus causes a similar condition in North America.

DISEASE MANAGEMENT

Fowl Cholera

Important Symptoms : In acute cases birds may die without showing any symptom. In less severe form breathing rapid-open beak, feather ruffled, comb and wattle become cyanotic. There may be yellowish diarrhoea. In chronic form swollen comb and wattle, joints hot and painful. In duck acute haemorrhagic enteritis and oozing of blood from oral cavity noticed. Sudden death will be occurring.

Specimens to be Collected : Blood smear from ailing bird, spleen, liver, lung etc. from sacrificed or dead bird in separate cover (on ice), long bones from putrefied carcass in charcoal packing. In chronic case smear from wattle.

Diagnosis : Demonstration of organism in blood smear, isolation of organism from internal organs, isolation of the organism from long bone, in chronic case it is difficult to demonstrate the organism in blood. Smear from wattle is used, biological method using pigeon.

Control/ Treatment

Treatment: Sulpha drugs and TMP combination, Enrofloxacin are effective. Drugs like Flamequin, Ampicillin, Chloramphenicol, Chlortetracycline and Novobiocin are also used.

- Killed vaccine
- Formalin's vaccines with adjuvant: 1 ml s/c.

PARATYPHOID INFECTION

Important Symptoms

Chicks hatched from infected egg, moribund or dead chick may be seen in the incubator. Sometimes disease is not seen for 5-10 days. Peak mortality during second or third week. Affected birds may exhibit a shrill cry when voiding excreta, which is white or greenish brown. Infection spread within the flock for a long time without any distinct signs. Reduction in egg production, fertility and hatchability.

Specimens to be Collected

Two ailing birds Internal organs in sterile vials, by special messenger on ice.

Diagnosis

Isolation and identification of organism, clinical observation and autopsy findings, serological tests.

Control/ Treatment

Furazlidone, injectable gentamicin, spectinomycin, and sodium nalidixate are the drugs of choice. Bacterin and attenuated live vaccines are used.

COLLIBACILLOSIS

Important Symptoms

In acute form, symptoms resemble fowl cholera or fowl typhoid.

Specimens to be Collected

Ailing bird or internal organs in sterile containers through special messenger on ice.

Diagnosis

Symptoms, isolation and identification of organism, PM lesions, pericarditis, peritonitis, air saculitis, perihepatitis, septicaemic carcass with liver, spleen, lung, kidney dark and congested.

Control/ Treatment

Faecal contamination of hatching eggs reduced by fumigating or disinfecting eggs within 2 hours of laying. Antibiotic administration after studying the antibiogram.

Furazolidone is fed (0.04 per cent) for 10 days and chlortetracycline in water (600 mg/5 L) for 5 days. Inactivated vaccine from 02:K1 and 078:KSO strains are effective. For ducks, inactivated vaccine prepared from 078 strains is effective.

INFECTIOUS CORYZA

Important Symptoms

Affects upper respiratory tract, sero mucoid nasal and occular discharges and facial oedema, conjunctivitis with closed eyes.

Specimens to be Collected

Ailing bird or trachea and lungs in sterile containers on ice.

Diagnosis

Isolation and identification.

Control/ Treatment

Sulpha drugs plus TMP, streptomycin, tetracycline, chloramphenicol, quinolone 2nd generation.

CHRONIC RESPIRATORY DISEASE (CRD)

Important Symptoms

Nasal discharge, shaking of head, coughing, swelling of the orbital sinuses and tracheal rales. Loss of weight, reduction in egg production and fertility, mortality low.

Specimens to be Collected

Ailing bird or trachea, air sac, turbinate and lung in sterile container from dead bird. Diagnosis Symptoms, isolation and identification of organism, rapid serum plate test, HI test, ELISA.

Control/ Treatment

Chlortetracycline, tylosin, streptomycin, erythromycin or lincomycin can be tried. But some strains are resistant to tylosin, streptomycin, erythromycin or spiromycin. Dipping of egg prior to hatching in tylosin or chlortetracycline is advised for controlling the infection.

- MG bacterin with oil emulsion adjuvant.
- Live vaccine F strain of MG can be used.

GANGRENOUS DERMATITIS

Important Symptoms

Varying degree of depression, in coordination, leg weakness, ataxia, dark moist areas of skin devoid of feathers, overlying wings, breast, abdomen and leg, extensive blood tinged edema with or without gas is present beneath the affected skin.

Specimens to be Collected

Ailing birds, swab collected from affected area.

Diagnosis

Clinical symptoms and lesions, isolation and identification of organism.

Control/ Treatment

No treatment is completely successful. Chlortetracycline, Oxytetracycline, Bacitracin, penicillin, copper sulphate in drinking water. Furaxone in feed

PSITTACOSIS/ORNITHOSIS

Important Symptoms

Ruffled plumage, nasal discharge, watery greenish diarrhea, pasting of feathers, wasting of pectoral muscles, nervous symptoms, respiratory symptoms.

Specimens to be Collected

Two ailing birds, impression smears from cut surfaces of liver, spleen, air sac impression smears.

Diagnosis

Clinical symptoms, P.M.findings, microscopical examination, impression smears, after modified ZN staining isolation and identification of the organism, CFT.

Control/ Treatment

Broad-spectrum antibiotics, chlortetracycline 500-800 g/tonne of feed for 3 weeks. Doxycycline also tried.

VIRAL CAUSED DISEASES

Fowlpox in Chickens and Turkeys

Fowlpox is a slow-spreading viral infection of chickens and turkeys characterized by proliferative lesions in the skin (cutaneous form) that progress to thick scabs and by lesions in the upper GI and respiratory tracts (diphtheritic form). It is seen worldwide.

Etiology and Epidemiology

The large DNA virus (an avipoxvirus, family Poxviridae) is highly resistant and may survive for several years in dried scabs. Field and vaccine strains have only minor differences in their genomic profiles, although the strains can be differentiated to some extent by restriction endonuclease analysis, and immunoblotting.

Recently, molecular analyses of vaccine and field strains of fowlpox viruses have shown some significant differences. The virus is present in large numbers in the lesions and is usually transmitted by contact through abrasions of the skin.

Skin lesions (scabs) shed from the recovering birds in poultry houses can become a source of aerosol infection. Mosquitos and other biting insects may serve as mechanical vectors. Transmission within flocks is rapid when mosquitos are plentiful. Some affected birds may become carriers, and the disease may be reactivated by stress (e.g., moulting) or by immunosuppression due to other infections. The disease tends to persist for extended periods in multiple-age poultry complexes.

Clinical Findings

Only a few birds develop lesions at one time. Lesions are prominent in some birds and may significantly decrease flock performance. The cutaneous form is characterized by nodular lesions on various parts of the unfeathered skin of chickens and on the head and upper neck of turkeys. Generalized lesions of feathered skin may also be seen.

In some cases, lesions are limited chiefly to the feet and legs. The lesion is initially a raised, blanched, nodular area that enlarges, becomes yellowish, and progresses to a thick, dark scab. Multiple lesions usually develop and often coalesce. Lesions in various stages of development may be found on the same bird. Localization around the nostrils may cause nasal discharge.

Cutaneous lesions on the eyelids may cause complete closure of one or both eyes. In the diphtheritic form, lesions develop on the mucous membranes of the mouth, esophagus, pharynx, larynx, and trachea (wetpox or fowl diphtheria).

Occasionally, lesions are seen almost exclusively in one or more of these sites. Caseous patches firmly adherent to the mucosa of the larynx and mouth or proliferative masses may develop. Mouth lesions interfere with feeding. Tracheal lesions cause difficulty in respiration and may simulate infectious laryngotracheitis in chickens. Laryngeal and tracheal lesions in chickens must be differentiated from those of laryngotracheitis.

Often, the course of the disease in a flock is protracted. Extensive infection in a layer flock results in decreased egg production. Cutaneous infections alone ordinarily cause low or moderate mortality, and these flocks generally return to normal production after recovery. Mortality is usually high in the generalized or diphtheritic form.

Diagnosis

Cutaneous infections usually produce characteristic gross and microscopic lesions. When only small lesions are present, it is often difficult to distinguish them from abrasions caused by fighting. Microscopic examination of affected tissues stained with H&E reveals eosinophilic cytoplasmic inclusion bodies. Cytoplasmic inclusions are also detectable by fluorescent antibody and immunohistochemical methods.

The elementary bodies in the inclusion bodies can be detected in smears from lesions stained by the Gimenez method. Viral particles with typical poxvirus morphology can be demonstrated by negative-staining electron microscopy as well as in ultrathin sections of the lesions. The virus can be isolated by inoculating chorioallantoic membrane of developing chicken embryos, susceptible birds, or cell cultures of avian origin. Chicken embryos (9-12 days old) are the preferred and most convenient host for virus isolation.

Field isolates and vaccine strains of fowlpox virus can be compared by restriction endonuclease analysis of viral genomes. This method is useful for comparing closely related DNA genomes. However, because of the large size of the genome, minor differences are difficult to detect by this method. Detailed genetic analysis reveals differences between vaccine strains and field strains responsible for outbreaks of fowlpox in previously vaccinated chicken flocks. While vaccine strains of fowlpox virus contain remnants of long terminal repeats of reticuloendotheliosis virus (REV), most field strains contain full- length REV in their genome. Nucleic acid probes derived from cloned genomic fragments of fowlpox virus can also be used for diagnosis. This procedure is especially useful for differentiation of the diphtheritic form of fowlpox (involving the trachea) from infectious laryngotracheitis.

PCR can be used to amplify genomic DNA sequences of various sizes using specific primers. This procedure is useful when an extremely small amount of viral DNA is present in the sample. PCR has been used effectively to differentiate field and vaccine strains of fowlpox virus. Recently, 2 monoclonal antibodies that recognize different fowlpox virus antigens have been developed. These monoclonal antibodies can be used for strain differentiation by immunoblotting. The complete sequence of the fowlpox virus genome has been identified recently and is useful in comparing the sequences of selected genes of other avian poxviruses.

Prevention and Treatment

Where pox is prevalent, chickens and turkeys should be vaccinated with live-embryo or cell-culture-propagated virus. The most widely used vaccines are attenuated fowlpox virus and pigeonpox virus isolates of high immunogenicity and low pathogenicity. A turkeypox vaccine has been developed to control pox in turkey flocks in which fowlpox vaccine has been ineffective.

This virus appears to be immunologically different from fowlpox virus. In high-risk areas, vaccination with an attenuated vaccine of cell-culture origin in the first few weeks of life and revaccination at 12-16 week is often sufficient. Health of birds, extent of exposure, and type of operation determine the timings of vaccinations.

Because the infection spreads slowly, vaccination is often useful in limiting spread in affected flocks if administered when <20 per cent of the birds have lesions. Because passive immunity may interfere with multiplication of vaccine virus, progeny from recently vaccinated or recently infected flocks should be vaccinated only after passive immunity has declined. Vaccinated birds should be examined 1 week later for swelling and scab formation ('take') at the site of vaccination. Absence of 'take' indicates lack of potency of vaccine, passive or acquired immunity, or improper vaccination. Revaccination with another serial lot of vaccine may be indicated.

Naturally infected or vaccinated birds develop humoral as well as cell- mediated immune responses. Humoral immune responses can be measured by ELISA or virus neutralization tests.

Infectious Bronchitis

Infectious bronchitis is an acute, rapidly spreading, viral disease of chickens characterized by respiratory signs, decreased egg production, and poor egg quality. Some strains of the causative virus, infectious bronchitis virus (IBV), are nephropathogenic. The latter strains produce interstitial nephritis resulting in significant mortality. Infectious bronchitis is of major economic importance to commercial chicken producers worldwide.

Etiology and Epidemiology

IBV, a coronavirus, is worldwide in distribution and has numerous serotypes. Two or more serotypes may be seen simultaneously in one geographic region. IBV is shed by infected chickens in respiratory discharges and feces. The highly contagious virus is spread by airborne droplets, ingestion of contaminated feed and water, and contaminated equipment and clothng of caretakers. Naturally infected chickens and those vaccinated with live IBV may intermittently shed virus for many weeks or even months. Virus infection in layers and breeders occurs cyclically as immunity declines or on exposure to different serotypes.

Clinical Findings

Signs occur after an incubation period of 18-48 hr. Spread to other birds is rapid, and morbidity may be nearly 100 per cent. The nature and severity of the disease are influenced by the age and immune status of the flock and virulence of the causal strain. Young chickens cough, sneeze, and have tracheal rales for 10-14 days. Wet eyes and dyspnea may be seen, and facial swelling may also occur ccasionally, particularly with concurrent bacterial infection of the sinuses. In broiler chickens, IBV infection is a major cause of poor feed conversion, reduced growth rate, and condemnation of meat at processing. Nephropathogenic strains can produce interstitial nephritis with high mortality (up to 60 per cent) in young chickens. In most outbreaks, however, mortality is 5 per cent, although secondary bacterial infections may cause higher losses.

In layers, egg production may drop 5-50 per cent, and eggs are often misshapen, thin-shelled, and contain watery albumen. Egg production and egg quality generally return to near normal levels in most birds on recovery.

Lesions

Respiratory tract lesions include mucoid exudate in the trachea and bronchi, generally without hemorrhage. Caseous plugs may be found in the trachea of young birds. Air sacs are thickened and opaque. Secondary bacterial infections in meat-type birds, especially with coliform bacteria, produce caseous airsacculitis, perihepatitis, and pericarditis. Nephropathogenic strains produce swollen, pale kidneys, with tubules and ureters distended with urates. In layers, urolithiasis is associated with virus infection and certain dietary factors.

Diagnosis

Diagnosis cannot be based solely on clinical signs because of similarities to mild respiratory forms of Newcastle disease, laryngotracheitis, and infectious coryza. Seroconversion or a rise in IBV antibody titer shown by ELISA, hemagglutination inhibition, or virus neutralization tests can be used for diagnosis given a history of respiratory disease or reduced egg production. A definitive diagnosis is generally based on virus isolation and identification.

Virus can be isolated by inoculation of bacteria-free tissue homogenates of trachea, cecal tonsils, and kidneys into 9-to 11-day-old chicken embryos. Several blind passages of the virus may be necessary for isolation of some field strains. The virus produces embryo stunting, curling, and urate deposits in the mesonephros, with variable mortality. Because the virus exhibits great antigenic variation, the serotype should be identified if possible.

Serotypes are conventionally identified with the aid of known serotype- specific chicken antisera in the virus neutralization test. However, the virus neutralization test is expensive, time consuming, and not readily available; therefore, it is not commonly used. A limited number of serotype-specific monoclonal antibodies (MAb) have been developed for serotyping purposes.

However, direct application of MAb-based immuno-histochemical procedures for detection of viral antigen in infected chicken tissues is not considered dependable because of the low concentration of the antigen in the tissues. The MAb have been best used after the virus is propagated by passage in chicken embryos, in which case the virus can be detected in the cells associated with the chorioallantoic membranes by immunofluorescence or immunoperoxidase staining, or in the allantoic fluid by ELISA.

Analyses of the viral genome for the purpose of identifying the virus serotype are now commonly used. These methods are based on the application of reverse transcriptase PCR (RT-PCR), using-specific oligonucleotide primers, to produce DNA copies of IBV genes, usually of the S1 part of the spike glycoprotein gene.

Subsequently, the RT-PCR product is subjected to restriction fragment length polymorphism (RFLP) or analysed by nucleotide sequencing. For RFLP, the RT-PCR product is digested with a set of specific restriction endonucleases, and the digested nucleic acid fragments are separated by gel electrophoresis. The specific pattern of their separation in the gel is compared with those of the standard strains for identification.

Control

No available medication alters the course of the disease, although antibiotic therapy may reduce mortality due to secondary infections. Increasing the temperature in the poultry house and under the hover by 5-10°F (3-5°C) may lower mortality. Attenuated vaccines used for immunization may produce mild respiratory signs. Live vaccines are initially given to chicks 1-14 days old by spray, drinking water, or eyedrop. Revaccination is common. Live or adjuvanted killed vaccines are sometimes used in breeders and layers to prevent egg production losses.

Many serotypes are recognized, and a number of new or variant serotypes have been reported, which pose problems in immunization and diagnosis. If possible, selection of vaccine should be based on knowledge of the prevalent serotype(s) on the premises. The most commonly used live vaccines in the USA contain strains of IBV serotypes Massachusetts, Connecticut, and Arkansas. Vaccination with selected variant serotypes is practiced in some areas. Outbreaks with mortality due to nephritis have been associated with several variant strains in Australia and the USA. Infection with standard as well as variant serotypes have been associated with egg production losses in vaccinated layer flocks.

Infectious Bronchitis (Ib)

This infection, probably the commonest respiratory disease of chickens, was first described in the USA (N. Dakota, 1931). Its affects vary with: the virulence of the virus; the age of the bird; prior vaccination; maternal immunity (young birds); and complicating infections (Mycoplasma, E. coli, Newcastle disease). Morbidity may vary 50-100 per cent and mortality 0-25 per cent, depending on secondary infections. The cause is a Coronavirus that is antigenically highly variable; new sero-types continue to emerge. About eight sero-groups are recognised by sero-neutralization. Typing by haemagglutination-inhibition is also used. These differences are due to structural differences in the spike proteins (S1 fraction).

Infection is via the conjunctiva or upper respiratory tract with an incubation period of 18-36 hours. The infection is highly contagious and spreads rapidly by contact, fomites or aerosol. Some birds/viral strains can be carriers to 1 year. The virus, which may survive 4 weeks in premises, is sensitive to solvents, heat (56°C for 15 mins), alkalis, disinfectants (Formal 1 per cent for 3 mins). Poor ventilation and high density are predisposing factors.

Signs

- Depression.
- Huddling.
- Loss of appetite.
- Coughing, gasping, dyspnoea.
- Wet litter.
- Diarrhoea.
- Diuresis.

Post-mortem Lesions

- Mild to moderate respiratory tract inflammation.
- Tracheal oedema.
- Tracheitis.
- Airsacculitis.
- Caseous plugs in bronchi.
- Kidneys and bronchi may be swollen and they and the ureters may have urates.

Diagnosis

Tentative diagnosis is based on clinical sgns, lesions and serology. Definitive diagnosis is based on viral isolation after 3-5 passages in chick embryo, HA negative, with typical lesions, flourescent antibody positive and ciliostasis in tracheal organ culture.

Differentiate from Newcastle disease (lentogenic and mesogenic forms), mycoplasmosis, vaccinal reactions, Avian Influenza and Laryngotracheitis.

Treatment

Sodium salicylate 1gm/litre (acute phase) where permitted-antibiotics to control secondary colibacillosis (q.v.).

Prevention

Live vaccines of appropriate sero-type and attenuation, possible reactions depending on virulence and particle size. Maternal immunity provides protection for 2-3 weeks. Humoral immunity appears 10-14 days post vaccination. Local immunity is first line of defence. Cell-mediated immunity may also be important.

Infectious Bursal Disease

Infectious bursal disease (also known as IBD, Gumboro Disease, Infectious Bursitis and Infectious Avian Nephrosis) is a highly contagious disease of young chickens caused by infectious bursal disease virus (IBDV), characterized by immunosuppression and mortality generally at 3 to 6 weeks of age. The disease was first discovered in Gumboro, Delaware in 1962. It is economically important to the poultry industry worldwide due to increased susceptibility to other diseases and negative interference with effective vaccination. In recent years, very virulent strains of IBDV (vvIBDV), causing severe mortality in chicken, have emerged in Europe, Latin America, South-East Asia, Africa and the Middle East. Infection is via the oro-fecal route, with affected bird excreting high levels of the virus for approximately 2 weeks after infection.

Virology

IBDV is a double stranded RNA virus that has a bi-segmented genome and belongs to the genus Avibirnavirus of family Birnaviridae. There are two distinct serotypes of the virus, but only serotype 1 viruses cause disease in poultry. At least six antigenic subtypes of IBDV serotype 1 have been identified by in vitro cross-neutralization assay. Viruses belonging to one of these antigenic subtypes are commonly known as variants, which were reported to break through high levels of maternal antibodies in commercial flocks, causing up to 60 to 100 per cent mortality rates in chickens. With the advent of highly sensitive molecular techniques, such as reverse transcription polymerase chain reaction (RT-PCR) and restriction fragment length polymorphism (RFLP), it became possible to detect the vvIBDV, to differentiate IBDV strains, and to use such information in studying the molecular epidemiology of the virus.

Viral Structure

The IBDV capsid protein exhibits structural domains that show homology to those of the capsid proteins of some positive-sense single-stranded RNA viruses, such as the nodaviruses and tetraviruses, as well as the T=13 capsid shell protein of the Reoviridae. The T=13 shell of the IBDV capsid is formed by trimers of VP2, a protein generated by removal of the C-terminal domain from its precursor, pVP2. The trimming of pVP2 is performed on immature particles as part of the maturation process. The other major structural protein, VP3, is a multifunctional component lying under the T=13 shell that influences the inherent structural polymorphism of pVP2. The virus-encoded RNA- dependent RNA polymerase, VP1, is incorporated into the capsid through its association with VP3. VP3 also interacts extensively with the viral dsRNA genome.

Pathogenesis

Clinical disease is associated to bird age with the greatest bursal mass, which occurs between 3 and 6 weeks of age. The greatest bursal mass is mostly a result of a large population of maturing IgM-bearing B-lymphocytes (lymphoblasts), the main target of infection. Young birds at around two to eight weeks of age that have highly active bursa of Fabricius are more susceptible to disease.

Birds over eight weeks are resistant to challenge and will not show clinical signs unless infected by highly virulent strains. Subclinical disease occurs in chickens infected before three weeks of age. At this age the B-lymphoblast population is smaller and the systemic effects are insufficient for generating clinical signs. However, the B-cell destruction is usually most severe in subclinically infected young, as virus will destroy a smaller population and most cells in one place (the bursa).

Clinical Signs

Disease may appear suddenly and morbidity typically reaches 100 per cent. In the acute form birds are prostrated, debilitated and dehydrated. They produce a watery diarrhea and may have swollen feces-stained vent. Most of the flock is recumbent and have ruffled feathers. Mortality rates vary with virulence of the strain involved, the challenge dose, previous immunity, presence of concurrent disease, as well as the flock's ability to mount an effective immune response. Immunosuppression of very young chickens, less than three weeks of age, is possibly the most important outcome and may not be clinically detectable (subclinical). In addition, infection with less virulent strains may not show overt clinical signs, but birds that have bursal atrophy with fibrotic or cystic follicles and lymphocytopenia before six weeks of age, may be susceptible to opportunistic infection and may die of infection by agents that would not usually cause disease in immunocompetent birds.

Diagnosis

A preliminary diagnosis can usually be made based on flock history, clinical signs and post-mortem (necropsy) examinations. However, definitive diagnosis can only be achieved by the specific detection and/ or isolation and characterization of IBDV. Immunofluorescence or immunohistochemistry tests, based on anti-IBDV labelled antibodies, or in-situ hybridization, based on labelled complementary cDNA sequence probe, are useful for the specific detection of IBDV in infected tissues.

RT-PCR was designed for the detection of IBDV genome, such as VP1 coding gene, with the possibility of PCR product sequences be determined for genetically comparing isolates and producing phylogenetic trees. Serological tests such as agar gel precipitation and ELISA, for detecting antibodies, are used for monitoring vaccine responses and might be additional information for diagnosis of infection of unvaccinated flocks.

Necropsy examination will usually show changes in the bursa of Fabricius such as swelling, oedema, haemorrhage, the presence of a jelly serosa transudate and eventually, bursal atrophy. Pathological changes, especially haemorrhages, may also be seen in the skeletal muscle, intestines, kidney and spleen.

Treatment and Control

Peri-focal vaccination may not be effective for the combat of an outbreak, due to the rapidity of wild-IBDV spreading. Passive immunity may protect against challenge with homologous IBDV, as does previous infection with homologous avirulent strains. Breeder flocks may be immunised against IBD so that they would transfer protective antibodies to their progenies, such as broiler and pullet chicks. Low-attenuated vaccine strains may cause damage to the bursa of Fabricius and immunosuppression in susceptible chicks. Biosecurity with adequate restriction to farm visitation and distancing from other flocks. Post outbreak hygiene measures may not be effective as the virus can survive for long periods in both housing and water.

Lymphoid Leucosis

Lymphoid leukosis occurs worldwide in chickens and some exotic birds. It usually affects birds of 16 weeks or older. Avian leucosis viruses are RNA retroviruses. There are 10 viral subgroups (A-J). Type A and J are most important. Vertically transmitted some horizontal transmission at young age in case of intensive contact.

Causes of Lymphoid Leukosis

The subgroup virus was commonly found in broiler breeders around 1994-1999. Nowadays, it is hardly seen due to severe eradication programmes at pedigree level. Osteopetrosis occurs in broiler-age birds. Lymphoid leukosis virus is an RNA virus in the family of retroviruses. Ten viral subgroups (A-J) are known. Avian leucosis viruses (ALVs) were common around the world, because they are transmitted through the eggs of common commercial breeders.

Mode of Transmission

It spreads through the egg (transovarian). It is a ubiquitous organism in commercial poultry flocks. There is some lateral transmission with congenitally infected chickens.

Effects of Lymphoid Leukosis

Signs include paleness, emaciation, weakness and inappetence. The abdomen is enlarged and feathers are sometimes spotted with urates and bile. The feed/gain ratio is decreased. Increased culls and decreased egg production occurs.

Post-mortem Lesions

Peripheral nerves are never involved. Bursae are always enlarged and may contain nodular tumours. Visceral tumours are soft, smooth and glistening. Tumours may be nodular, military or diffuse. Tumours are common in gonads, lungs, liver, spleen, heart, kidney, mesentery and bone marrow. The skin is never affected and skeletal muscles often contain tumours. Eyes are never affected. Bone sometimes contains tumours (especially with J virus). The blood often contains tumours (especially with J virus). Fat tumours are common (Liposarcoma).

Diagnosis of Lymphoid Leukosis

Tumours in adult birds are characteristic for this disease. Liposarcoma or myeloid tumour (J virus) is also characteristic. ELISA tests are available to detect both the antigen (P27) and the antibodies against J virus. Histopathology an ovoid nucleus and a finer, more delicate chromatin network. PCR test is used to select out J virus positive broiler breeder grandparent stock. ELISA test use specific serum to determine the presence of the organism in serum, vaginal swab or egg albumin. PCR test used for J virus. Different diagnosis: E. coli, Aspergillus, MD, tuberculosis, erythroblastosis and myelobastosis.

The tumours are grossly distinct from those caused by other ALVs. However, the definitive diagnosis is based on virological isolation or histologic observation of the tumour cells. The myeloid cells can be differentiated from other tumour cell types by a trained histopathologist.

Marek's Disease

Mareks' disease occurs worldwide in chickens (all breeds), pheasants, turkeys and occasionally quail. It usually affects birds under 16 weeks, but birds can die near the onset of egg production. Marek's disease virus is a cell- associated herpes virus containing double-stranded DNA, of which there are three serotypes. Only serotype 1.

Causes of Mareks' disease

It was named after a Hungarian pathologist (Josef Marek) and also because it caused paralysis is chickens, which use to be reared on the range (range paralysis). It affects chickens (all breeds), occasionally pheasants and quail. It occurs worldwide in commercial flocks. Disease is chronic. It takes 4-6 weeks for tumours to form. Classical type (nervous form) is common in white layers between 6-16 weeks. Visceral type with tumours in various internal organs usually occurs between 16-35 weeks. Infection takes place at very young age, but birds can die of Marek's disease (MD) near the onset of egg production.

It is caused by a cell-associated Herpes virus containing double-stranded DNA. It has hexagonal naked particles or nucleocapsids of 85 or 100 nm. Marek's disease viruses and Marek's disease vaccines are classified into 3 serotypes. Serotype 1 viruses can be oncogenis (cause tumours).

Mode of Transmission

It is spread by contaminated litter, dust, down or air-borne (bird to bird). Feather (dust or dander) epithelium contains virus. There is an incubation period of 2 weeks for virus shed and for clinical signs from 3-6 weeks.

Syndromes

There are six syndromes known to occur after infection with Marek's disease. These syndromes may overlap.

- ClassicalMarek'sdiseaseorneurolymphomatosiscausesasymmetric paralysis of one or more limbs. With vagus nerve involvement, difficulty breathing or dilation of the crop may occur. Besides lesions in the peripheral nerves, there are frequently lymphomatous infiltration/tumours in the skin, skeletal muscle, visceral organs. Organs that are commonly affected include the ovary, spleen, liver, kidneys, lungs, heart, proventriculus and adrenals.
- Acute Marek's disease is an epidemic in a previously uninfected or unvaccinated flock, causing depression, paralysis, and death in a large number of birds (up to 80 per cent). The age of onset is much earlier than the classic form; birds are four to eight weeks old when affected. Infiltration into multiple organs/tissue is observed.
- Ocular lymphomatosis causes lymphocyte infiltration of the iris (making the iris turn grey), anisocoria, and blindness.
- Cutaneous Marek's disease causes round, firm lesions at the feather follicles.
- Atherosclerosis is induced in experimentally infected chickens.
- Immunosuppression–Impairment of the T-lympho-cytes prevent competent immunological response against pathogenic challenge and the affected birds become more susceptible to disease conditions such as coccidiosis and 'Escherichia coli' infection. Furthermore, without stimulation by cell-mediated immunity, the humoral immunity conferred by the B-cell lines from the Bursa of Fabricius also shuts down, thus resulting in birds that are totally immuno-compromised.

Diagnosis

Diagnosis of lymphoid tumors in poultry is complicated due to multiple etiological agents capable of causing very similar tumors. It is not uncommon that more than one avian tumour virus can be present in a chicken, thus one must consider both the diagnosis of the disease/tumors (pathological diagnosis) and of the virus (etiological diagnosis). A step-wise process has been proposed for diagnosis of Marek's disease which includes (1) history, epidemiology, clinical observations and gross necropsy, (2) characteristics of the tumour cell, and (3) virological characteristics The demonstration of peripheral nerve enlargement along with suggestive clinical signs in a bird that is around three to four months old (with or without visceral tumors) is highly suggestive of Marek's Disease.

Histological examination of nerves reveals infiltration of pleomorphic neo- plastic and inflammatory lymphocytes. Peripheral neuropathy should also be considered as a principal rule out in young chickens with paralysis and nerve enlargement without visceral tumors, especially in nerves with interneuritic edema and infiltration of plasma cells is confirmatory. It reveals large lymphoblasts in toumours. Lymphoblastshave disease but further testing is required for confirmation. This is done through histological demonstration of lymphomatous infiltration into the affected tissue. A range of leukocytes can be involved, including lymphocytic cell lines such as large lymphocyte, lymphoblast, primitive reticular cells and occasional plasma cells as well as macrophage and plasma cells. The T-cells are involved in the malignancy, showing neo-plastic changes with evidence of mitosis. The lymphomatous infiltrates need to be differentiated from other conditions that affect poultry including Lymphoid Leukosis and Reticuloendotheliosis, as well as an inflammatory event associated with hyperplastic changes of the affected tissue.

Key clinical signs as well as gross and microscopic features that are most useful for differentiating Marek's disease from Lymphoid Leukosis and Reticuloendotheliosis include (1) Age: MD can affect birds at any age, including <16 weeks of age; (2) Clinical signs: Frequent wing and leg paralysis; (3) Incidence: >5 per cent in unvaccinated flocks; (4) Potential nerve enlargement; (5) Interfollicular tumors in the Bursa of Fabricius; (6) CNS involvement; (7) Lymphoid proliferation in skin and feather follicles; (8) Pleomorphic lymphoid cells in nerves and tumors; (9) T-cell lymphomas. In addition to gross pathology and histology, other advanced procedures used for a definitive diagnosis of Marek's disease include immunohistochemistry to identify cell type and virus-specific antigens, standard and quantitative PCR for identification of the virus, virus isolation to confirm infections and serology to confirm/exclude infections.

Prevention

Vaccination is the only known method to prevent the development of tumors when chickens are infected with the virus. However, administration of vaccines does not prevent transmission of the virus, i.e., the vaccine is non- sterilizing. However, it does reduce the amount of virus shed in the dander and hence reduce horizontal spread of the disease. Marek's Disease does not spread vertically. The vaccine was introduced in 1970 and the scientist credited with its development is Dr. Ben Roy Burmester.

Before that, Marek's disease caused substantial revenue loss in the poultry industries of the United States and the United Kingdom. The vaccine can be administered to one day old chicks through sub-cutaneous inoculation or by in-ovo vaccination when the eggs are transferred from the incubator to the hatcher. In-ovo vaccination is the preferred method, as it does not require handling of the chicks and can be done rapidly by automated methods. Immunity develops within two weeks.

The vaccine originally contained the antigenically similar turkey herpesvirus, which is serotype 3 of MDV. However, because vaccination does not prevent infection with the virus, the Marek's Disease virus has evolved increased virulence and resistance to this vaccine. As a result, current vaccines use a combination of vaccines consisting of HVT and gallid herpesvirus type 3 or an attenuated MDV strain, CVI988-Rispens.

Effects of Mareks' Disease

It causes increased susceptibility (immunosuppression) to other diseases. Signs include weak, pale, off feed, diarrhoea, poor performance, culls and blindness. In white leghorn type birds, Classical Marek is common. There is paralysis or perisis (partial paralysis). There can be unilateral or bilateral paralysis of wings and legs, mortality, tumours and central nervous system signs (tremors). One leg stretches forward and the other backwards due to leg paralysis.

Postmortem Lesions

The peripheral nerves are often enlarged (vagus, sacaral, sciatic and brachial) with a loss of striations. They can also have grey or yellow discolouration and be edematous (fluid filled). The bursae are sometimes enlarged with tumours, but most often is strophic. There are enlarged organs (gonads, spleen, heart, lungs, liver, kidneys, proventriculus, intestines etc.) with focal to nodular, palpable tumours. The skeletal muscles have tumours. The eye (iris and pupil) may have diffuse depigmentation, diffuse bluish fading or diffuse grey opacity of the iris. The pupil may be irregular and tiny.

Diagnosis of Mareks' disease

The diagnosis is by observation of gross tumours in immature birds. Ocular or skin leucosis and nerve involvement are diagnostic for MD. Histopathologically, small to medium lymphocytes comprise tumours. Lymphoid cells occur in peripheral nerves. It simulates riboflavin deficiency, lymphoid leucosis, reticuloendotheliosis and colibacillosis.

Treatment and Control of Mareks' Disease

Prevention : Vaccinate (HVT-serotype 3 alone, or HVT and SB1-serotype 2) chicks at day-old subcutaneously in the hatchery. Some injections are done at 18 days or embryonation (in ovo). HVT and SB1 are used for broiler breeders and white leghorns at full dosage. HVT is used alone or HVT and SB1 at 1/3-1/4 dosage for broilers if they are to be kept over 50 days, although broiler vaccination is common in the US.

SB1 may cause immunosuppression and increase leucosis is some Leghorn strains. HVT = Herpes virus of turkeys. SB1 = S (susceptible strain) and B1 (pen B1). HVT + SB1 or HVT + Rispens vaccine can be used. Rispens strain (Serotype 1) may be used alone or in combination with HVT. Outside the USA, Rispens strain is the most commonly used vaccine, usually given by intramuscular injection at day old. In areas with a high infection risk bivalent vaccine (Rispens + HVT) is used.

Treatment

None.

Newcastle Disease

Poultry and many other bird species. It is a worldwide problem that presents primarily as a respiratory disease, but depression, nervous manifestations, or diarrhea may be the predominant clinical form. Mortality is variable. Occurrence of a virulent form of the disease is reportable and may result in trade restrictions.

Etiology and Pathogenesis

Newcastle disease is caused by an RNA virus, Newcastle disease virus (NDV), synonymous with avian paramyxovirus-1 which is in the genus Avulavirus, family Paramyxoviridae. Isolates are classified into 1 of 3 virulence groups by chicken embryo and chicken inoculation as virulent (velogenic), moderately virulent (mesogenic), or of low virulence (lentogenic). Lentogenic strains are used widely as live vaccines in healthy chickens. Clinical manifestations vary from high morbidity and mortality to asymptomatic infections. The severity of an infection is dependent on virus virulence and the age, immune status, and susceptibility of the host species. Chickens are the most and waterfowl the least susceptible of domestic poultry.

Epidemiology and Transmission

Virulent NDV strains are endemic in poultry in most of Asia, Africa, and some countries of North, Central, and South America. Other countries, including the USA and Canada, are free of those strains and maintain that status with import restrictions and eradication by destroying diseased poultry. Cormorants, pigeons, and imported psittacine species have also been sources of virulent NDV infections of poultry. Low virulence NDV is prevalent in poultry and wild birds, especially waterfowl. Infection of domestic poultry with low virulence NDV contributes to lower productivity.

Infected birds shed virus in exhaled air, respiratory discharges, and feces. Virus is shed during incubation, during the clinical stage, and for a varying but limited period during convalescence. Virus may also be present in eggs laid during clinical disease and in all parts of the carcass during acute virulent infections. Chickens are readily infected by aerosols and by ingesting contaminated water or food. Infected chickens are the primary source of virus, but other domestic and wild birds may be sources of NDV. Transfer of virus, especially in infective feces, by the movement of people and contaminated equipment is the main method of spread between poultry flocks.

Clinical Findings

Onset is rapid, and signs appear throughout the flock within 2-12 days (average 5) after aerosol exposure. Spread is slower if the fecal-oral route is the primary means of transmission, particularly for caged birds. Young birds are the most susceptible.

Observed signs depend on whether the infecting virus has a predilection for respiratory, digestive, or nervous systems. Respiratory signs of gasping, coughing, sneezing, and rales predominate in low virulence infections. Nervous signs of tremors, paralyzed wings and legs, twisted necks, circling, clonic spasms, and complete paralysis may accompany, but usually follow, the respiratory signs in neurotropic velogenic disease.

Nervous signs with diarrhea are typical in pigeons, and nervous signs are frequently seen in cormorants and exotic bird species. Respiratory signs with depression, watery-greenish diarrhea, and swelling of the tissues of the head and neck are typical of the most virulent form of the disease, viscerotropic velogenic Newcastle disease (VVND, also called exotic Newcastle disease), although nervous signs may also be seen. Varying degrees of depression and inappetence are observed. A partial or complete cessation of egg production may occur. Eggs may be abnormal in colour, shape, or surface, and have watery albumen. Mortality is variable but can be as high as 100 per cent.

Lesions

Remarkable gross lesions are usually observed only with VVND. Petechiae may be seen on the serous membranes; hemorrhages of the proventricular mucosa and intestinal serosa are accompanied by multifocal, necrotic hemorrhagic areas on the mucosal surface of the intestine, especially at lymphoid foci such as cecal tonsils. Splenic necrosis and hemorrhage and edema around the thymus may also be observed. In contrast, the lesions in birds infected with lower virulence NDV strains may be limited to congestion and mucoid exudates seen in the respiratory tract with opacity and thickening of the air sacs. Secondary bacterial infections will increase the severity of the respiratory lesions.

Diagnosis

Diagnosis may be confirmed by isolation of a hemagglutinating virus identified by inhibition with Newcastle disease antiserum. A rise in hemagglutination-inhibition antibodies in paired serum samples also confirms the disease. The acute form should be differentiated from highly pathogenic avian influenza (Avian Influenza: Introduction).

Virulence of an isolate is established by the rapidity of killing day-old chicks inoculated by the intracerebral route, the intracerebral pathogenicity index, or by the presence of a specified amino acid motif at the cleavage site of the fusion protein (F) precursor (FO). Reference laboratories use monoclonal antibodies to detect antigenic differences and nucleotide sequence analysis to detect genetic differences for comparison of isolates from different outbreaks and to identify the source of those infections.

Prevention

Live lentogenic vaccines, chiefly B1 and LaSota strains, are widely used and typically administered to poultry by mass application in drinking water or by spray. Alternatively, individual administration is via the nares or conjunctival sac. Healthy chicks are vaccinated as early as day 1-4 of life. However, delaying vaccination until the second or third week avoids maternal antibody interference with an active immune response. Mycoplasma, some other bacteria, and other viruses affecting the respiratory tract, if present, may act synergistically with some vaccines to aggravate the vaccine reaction after spray administration.

Oil-adjuvanted inactivated vaccines are also used following live vaccine in breeders and layers and may be used alone in situations where use of live virus may be contraindicated. In countries where virulent NDV is endemic, a combination of live virus and inactivated vaccine can be used; or alternatively, if permitted by law, a live mesogenic strain vaccine may be used in older birds. The frequency of revaccination to protect chickens throughout life largely depends on the risk of exposure and virulence of the field virus challenge.

Zoonotic Risk

Newcastle disease viruses, whether virulent field viruses or live vaccine, can produce a transitory conjunctivitis in humans, but the condition has been limited primarily to laboratory workers and vaccination teams exposed to large quantities of virus. Before poultry vaccination was widely practiced, conjunctivitis from NDV infection occurred in crews eviscerating poultry in processing plants. The disease has not been reported in people who rear poultry or consume poultry products.

KINDS OF POULTRY VIRUS DISEASE

Ranikhet disease, also known in the West as Newcastle disease is a contagious and highly fatal daises of flows. In spite of the notable work done towards its control, this disease still ranks as one of the most serious virus diseases of poultry. The disease occurs in almost all countries and usually assumes a server form affecting birds of all ages. Mortality in flows varies from 50 to 100 per cent.

Ranikhet disease is largely a disease of flows, but it also effects turkeys, pigenosn, grows, ducks, geese, koel pheasants, guinea-flows, partridges and doves. hedgehogs have been suspected as reservoirs of the disease. The disease is also suspected to cause conjunctivitis among laboratory workers and persons handling infected birds.

Symptoms

The symptoms vary according to the age of the affected birds. The first symptoms usually observed in young birds are sneezing, gasping and often droopiness. It is in this stage of the disease that the manifestations rather closely resemble those of infections bronchitis. Within a short time after appearance of respiratory symptoms, deaths occur in a flock in quick succession and in increasing numbers from day to day.

Among growing birds and in adult sudden deaths occur in a dew instances, and are followed by a number of birds showing respiratory symptoms. The affected birds are full and depressed with ruffled feathers. These symptoms are accompanied by diarrhea, characterize by the passing of a watery stool with an offensive smell. There is profuse salivation. The saliva often accumulates in the mouth and obstructs respiration, which results in the production of gurgling disused birds may be soft-shelled and deformed. In turkeys the disease runs a very mild course. In adults, in particular, it may pass unnoticed except for some dullness, loss of appetite and other minor symptoms.

Treatment and Prevention

At present there is no effective treatment of any value. Proper housing and general good care are indicated in an effort to shorten the duration and severity of the infection.

An early recognition of the disease and application of struck sanitary measures are of great value in the control of the disease. Some important measures for its prevention are; slaughtering of all apparently ailing birds, segregating of in-contact in group of 10 to 15 each; removal of all infective materials such as droppings, residues of poultry cleanliness; and provision of separate attendants for each group of birds.

The poultry farm should be at a distance from place of traffic. All newly purchased birds should be kept in segregation from not less than 10 days before taking them into the farm. The poultry runs should be ploughed from time to time and lime applied thereon as a general disinfectant. As far as possible the pens and runs should be made inaccessible to free-flying birds by providing a barrier of wire-netting.

Control

Control of Ranikhet diseases can be effect with judicious application of sanitary and vaccination measures. The possibility of entry and spread of infection is considerably reduced through the maintenance of flock on deep little system and stopping all unauthorized entries, even of human beings, into the battery brooders. Disposal of fowl carcasses by burning or deep brutal to reduce the scope of carrion-eating birds like crows, kites and vultures perching near fowl pens or poultry farms helps to resume the hazards of this infection. Two types of vaccines are available in India, one for the adult birds an another for younger birds or body chicks.

The virus strain for Ranikeht disease vaccine used for adult birds age over weeks was evolved at the Indian veterinary Research Institute. The vaccine consists of freeze-dried virus grown in chick embryos. Vaccination of birds 6 weeks old and above confers immunity for 1 to 3 years.

Care should be taken to vaccinate bird's not carrying heavy coccidian infection. Birds with heavy worm infection or coccidiosis are not protected even with a good vaccine. There are sometimes complications side reactions following vaccination. There are sometimes complications side reactions following vaccination with 'Mukteswar' strain of Ranikhet disease vaccine. These consist on inco-ordination of limbs and sometimes paralysis in 1 to 3 per cent to the vaccinated birds. The reactions may become more acute if the birds are affected with roundworms, coccidiosis or are weak on account of malnutrition.

Table: Vaccination Programme for Layer Type Chicken

	Age	Disease	Vaccine	Route
1.	1 day	Marek's	HVT vaccine	I/M
2.	5-7 days	RD	Lasota/F	Occulonasal
3.	10-14 days	IBD	IBD Live	Drinking water
4.	24-28 days	IBD	IBD Live	Drinking water
5.	8th week	RD	R2B/RDVK	S/C
6.	16-18 week	RD	Killed/Live	S/C

Deworming

Birds should be dewormed starting from one week prior to R2B/RDVK vaccination and repeated at 3-week intervals so as to give a total of 4 dewormings before housing at 18 weeks of age. Piperazine compounds, albendazole, mebendazole etc. can be used against round worms. Against tape worms, Niclosamide, Praziquintel, Albendazole can be used. While medicating through drinking water, it should be done by mixing the required quantity of medicine in the quantity of water that chicks normally consume in 4 hours time (say approximately 6 litres per one hundred, 6 week-old chicks, per day). Additional water should be given only when all the medicated water is consumed by the chicks.

Ectoparasites

The birds should be dusted or dipped and houses fumigated as soon as there is indication of ectoparasites. The following may be used for dusting and dipping. Dipping should be avoided on rainy days. Head dipping has to be avoided.

1. Tick tox – synthetic pyrithrine compound. Dose – as per manufacturer's instructions
2. Butox – Deltamethrin compound. Dose – as per manufacturer's instructions.

In addition to these, general measures of sanitation such as keeping young stock away from adult stock, keeping the poultry houses and equipments clean, prohibiting visitors into the poultry house, proper disposal of dead birds, prevention of entry of rodents and other birds into the pen and periodical culling will greatly help in checking diseases.

□

3

Poultry Production and Poultry Preservation

POULTRY PRODUCTION

Using the word alternative in this context is a misnomer. Many types of poultry have been raised on pasture for hundreds of years. Pastured poultry production is used to describe a variety of production systems in which birds have access to pasture on a regular basis. Production systems vary widely from stationary houses with permanent yards to portable houses that are moved frequently to a new pasture. Additionally, birds may be allowed to free range in the pasture, most commonly seen in laying flocks or be confined to a portable house that is rotated throughout the pastures. There are no parameters for stocking rates on pastured poultry in the U.S.

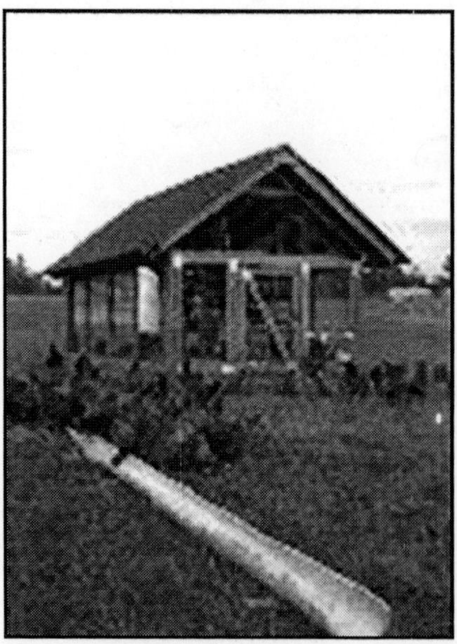

Fig: Free Range Laying Flock.

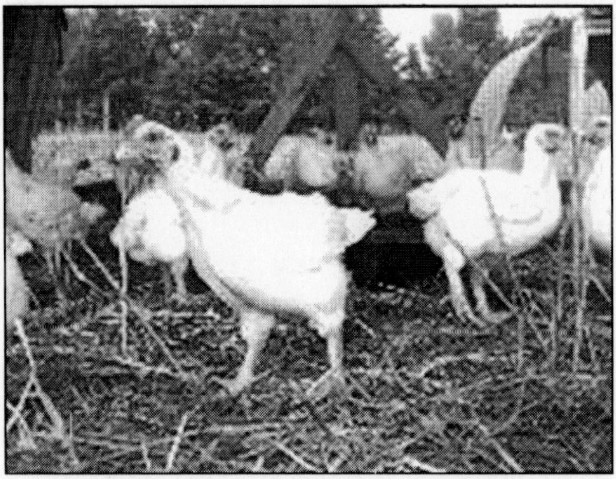

Fig: Cornish Cross Broiler Inside a Hoop House.

LIGHTING FOR ALTERNATIVE POULTRY PRODUCTION

Energy-Efficient Lighting for the Farm from the US National Sustainable Agriculture Information Service (ATTRA) provides an overview of energy-efficient lighting technology and explains how to select lighting options that are appropriate for the farm, including alternative poultry production.

Energy-efficient lighting options present farmers with new opportunities to reduce electricity costs and help manage farms sustainably. Cost-effective energy-efficient lighting can be used to improve productivity and safety, and reduce operating costs.

Supplemental lighting is normally used by alternative egg producers to maintain productivity, and sometimes for alternative broiler production in northern climates. Small layer flocks housed during late spring through mid- summer with daily access to the outdoors do not require supplemental light. Supplemental lighting is necessary for pullets to maintain production during late fall and winter as days shorten.

Poultry are very sensitive to three aspects of light: intensity of light (measured in footcandles), wavelength (measured in colour temperature), and day length (duration of light period). Research by Michael Darre and others has found that blue light wavelengths help calm birds; red wavelengths may be used to help reduce feather picking; blue-green wavelengths help maintain growth; and orange-red wavelength helps maintain reproduction.

The light intensity for layers should be enough to read a newspaper by and will vary with the poultry breed. Generally, 'warm' wavelength lamps of less than 3,000K in the red-orange spectrum are best for small flocks with outdoor access. The day length should never be extended past 16 hours or the longest day of the year.

Solar photovoltaic lighting provides a simple solution to maintaining egg production during shorter days. Solar lighting systems basically consist of a solar module, a deep-cycle battery, a charge controller, a 12V programmable timer, and an efficient DC lighting fixture with lamp. Energy-efficient LED basic low-voltage solar lighting system can be purchased online for less than $300 or as a kit.

To conserve energy and keep poultry healthy, use timers to switch lights on and off. Programmable timers must be 12V when used in conjunction with a 12V solar lighting system. Th ere are 12V timers available online as well as schematics to convert a household programmable thermostat to a 12V timer. Timers also ensure that birds receive a uniform number of light hours each day. Set timers to light in the morning instead of the evening to give birds a natural dusk and allow them to roost. Check timers at least once a week, and clean lamps if dust builds up. Lamps should be free of obstructions that cause shadows on the floor.

Baby chicks require additional light in their first 72 hours to help them find food and water. A low watt 'warm' lamp is recommended for every 200 square feet of floor space. (Hawes) The high heat from incandescent lamps may double as a brood light and heat source, although it may be more energy- efficient (and cost-effective) to use a separate heat source and a solar lighting system.

POULTRY PRODUCTION INDUSTRY

As poultry production is a prime example of a vertically integrated agricultural industry, with intensive rearing systems of birds of efficient feed conversion ratios and products of handy size and ready marketability, it is not surprising that it is currently showing the strongest growth in output of any category of meat. World-wide, it is a huge industry. Estimates of poultry populations. The largest increase in poultry populations between 1979 and 1989 are in N&C America, S America and Asia. As a general rule, poultry populations in developing countries are rising at a faster rate than in developed countries.

Table: World Population of Poultry in Selected Regions ('000's)

	1979	1987	1988	1989	% increase 79-89	% increase human pop 79-89
Africa	560	837	867	873	56	38
N&C America	758	1715	2089	2125	180	16
S America	552	843	896	961	74	22
Asia	2816	4347	4500	4702	67	22

Europe	1265	1373	1392	1394	10	3
Oceania	56	73	84	73	30	17
USSR	953	1174	1177	1207	27	10
Developed	3135	4362	4780	4810	53	8
Countries Developing	3826	6001	6226	6525	71	25
Countries World	6962	10364	11005	11335	63	20

Because poultry has a very short life cycle and poultry products are traded internationally, data on regional flock sizes are difficult to interpret. Estimates of world poultry meat production in metric tonnes.

The largest increase in poultry meat production took place in S America, particularly in the mid 1980's. The increase in developing countries has generally been higher than in developed countries but the impact is reduced because the increase in human population has been greater.

Poultry production is three times population growth in developed countries but only double population growth in less developed countries.

Table: Poultry meat production (1000 t)

	1979	1987	1988	1989	% Increase 79-89	% increase human pop 79-89
Africa	1090	1620	1658	1708	57	38
N&C America	9896	11026	11474	12087	22	16
S America	1608	9154	9480	10088	526	22
Asia	6350	7987	8304	8587	35	22
Europe	6812	8043	8237	8254	21	3
Oceania	283	439	468	460	63	17
USSR	2000	3127	3235	3250	62	10
Developed	19639	23386	24118	24731	26	8
Countries Developing	8400	12216	12795	13086	56	25
Countries World	28039	35603	36913	37817	35	20

POULTRY CONSUMPTION

Estimates of world poultry consumption are detailed in Table below. Levels of poultry consumption are increasing throughout the world and the increase in developing countries is about double the world average. This has been achieved through increased local production which has kept pace with demand.

Table: World poultry meat consumption (kg per head of human population)

	1979	1987	1988	1989	% increase 79-89	% increase human pop 79-89
Africa	2.49	3.00	2.94	2.90	16	38
N&C America	26.76	26.23	27.07	27.96	4	16
S America	6.58	32.1	32.43	33.81	414	22
Asia	2.68	2.92	2.97	3.04	13	22
Europe	13.37	15.19	15.39	15.52	16	3
Oceania	12.96	18.03	18.91	18.47	43	17
USSR	8.12	11.64	11.94	11.73	44	10
Developed	16.65	18.67	19.12	19.45	17	8
Countries Developing	2.77	3.35	3.41	3.42	23	25
Countries World	6.47	7.09	7.20	7.25	12	20

lamp work very well with solar modular. All of the components to build a or 12-60g per day depending on age and weight. Poultry products such as chicken have a high protein content. Table shows the per cent protein content of some common foods and their consumption. The table shows that the less developed countries appear to consume sufficient protein. A better interpretation would be that there is sufficient protein available for all to eat. In practice, protein distribution is skewed in Idc's so that some areas have plenty whereas others have very little.

Table: % Protein content and consumption of some common foods

Food type (Protein source)	% Protein	Developed	Consumption in kg dry matter/ head/yr 1989 Developing	World
Chicken	19			
Duck	11	3.70	0.65	1.38
Turkey	21			
Beef	21	5.68	0.83	2.00
Pork	25	8.14	1.87	3.36
Sheep	23	0.26	0.18	0.29
Fish	17	3.14	1.14	1.62
Milk	3.5	10.70	0.90	3.25
Egg	12.8	1.96	0.51	0.86
Rice	7.6	1.54	9.23	7.39
Wheat	8.4	26.1	9.68	13.70

Pulses	6	1.01	0.56	0.67
Groundnuts	25	0.49	1.27	1.09
Soya Beans	40	19.33	4.76	8.22
Potatoes	2.1	3.39	0.40	1.11
Total		85.44	31.98	43.56

Although this document concerns slaughter and processing for meat production, poultry are also kept for their eggs. Eggs are a highly versatile food containing many essential nutrients.

They are classified in the same protein food group as meat, poultry and fish. In developed countries per capita consumption of eggs has remained almost static over the last ten years but in less developed countries has risen by 37 per cent, about 1.5 times faster than population growth. This has been achieved through improvements in local production rather than increased importation. This indicates a sharp increase in poultry husbandry skills and readiness to undertake intensive production. The flocks used for both table and hatchery egg production are found in significant numbers and eventually end up at poultry processing plants.

The outlook for world poultry production is for continued strong growth. Poultry production is projected to continue to expand in N&C America and the EC. Further growth in Asia, particularly Thailand, is expected as a result of strong demand from Japan and the development of the EC market. Growing domestic demand in Brazil and China should result in higher production levels. In the old Soviet Bloc and eastern Europe, production is projected to fall as a result of reorganisation following market liberalisation. Demand in less developed countries will continue to grow at least apace with population.

Table: World consumption of hen eggs in shell (kg per head of human population)

	1979	1989	% increase 79-89	% increase human pop 79-89
Africa	1.97	2.35	19.27	38
N&C America	14.35	12.99	-9.46	16
S America	5.19	7.06	35.87	22
Asia	3.34	4.46	33.34	22
Europe	14.26	14.38	0.83	3
Oceania	11.74	9.51	-18.97	17
USSR	13.89	16.23	16.79	10
Developed Countries	15.06	15.34	1.86	8
Developing Countries	2.88	3.95	37.20	25
World	6.12	6.67	8.94	20

WORLDWIDE POULTRY MEAT PRODUCTION, CONSUMPTION FORECASTS

Visions of the year 2020 from various sources suggest that the world production of poultry meat will approach 122.5 million metric tons and that 72 million metric tons of eggs will be produced globally by then. The potential market size by that time is indicated by a projected growth of the global human population from 6 billion in 1999 and approximately 7 billion in 2011, to a total of 7.5 billion people in 2020.

With the projected increases in per-person consumption of poultry meat and eggs over the next decades, the global market's composition is forecast to change so that chicken rivals pork as the world's most popular meat.

Most of the extra demand for meat will be in the Asia-Pacific region, with large increases for a number of Asian countries.

In preparing the latest annual "Agricultural Outlook" publication on global prospects for the agriculture and food sectors, covering years 2011 to 2020, the Organisation for Economic Co-operation and Development, and the Food and Agriculture Organisation of the United Nations worked on the basis of a series of assumptions. These included that world economies would continue recovering from crisis, population growth would continue to slow and energy prices would trend upwards.

The groups also recognised that many of the drivers of high and volatile commodity prices - weather, yields, cereals stocks and energy prices - may themselves be more volatile in the future.

So while being cautiously optimistic that commodity prices would fall from the peaks of 2010 to 2011, the authors maintained the previously expressed view that agricultural commodity prices were likely to remain on a higher level during the next decade.

Slower Rise for Population

Nevertheless agricultural production and trade will continue to grow, the authors concluded, led by emerging economies where economic growth has resumed and appears to be resisting higher prices. All eyes at present are on the so-called BRIC countries of Brazil, Russia, India and China. After rising by almost 7.5 per cent in 2011, the BRIC countries' average annual economic growth, as measured by gross domestic product per person, has been projected to slow to 5.7 per cent in 2015 and 4.75 per cent in 2020, though still above the rates of other members of the developing countries group.

The annual growth rate of the world population, after averaging 1.2 per cent in the past decade, is expected to drop to 1.05 per cent between 2011 and 2020. The slowdown applies across all regions, said the OECD-FAO report, although more in developed rather than developing countries. Meanwhile the phenomenon of greater urbanisation will continue to reshape consumption patterns towards higher value processed products and convenience foods.

Firm demand, particularly from developing countries in Asia and Latin America, is forecast to boost the meat market in the decade ahead. FAO says world meat production will grow at an average rate of 1.8 per cent per year until 2020, adding some 60 million metric tons in the process, and that 78 per cent of the projected growth in meat supplies will involve production primarily of poultry and pig meat in the developing countries.

But the trade in poultry meat between countries will grow relatively slowly, at around 2 per cent per year, rather than the 4.7 per cent per year growth rate of exports seen in the past decade. The expectation is that the USA and Brazil will strengthen their dominance of world trade over the period so that, by 2020, the two countries account for nearly half of the additional export supply in world markets.

According to a European Commission report on prospects for agricultural markets, EU-27 poultry meat production could grow to 12.47 million metric tons in 2020, from under 12 million tons in 2011 and around 12.2 million tons in 2015. The uptake of poultry meat by European Union consumers seems set to grow from the current 23.4 kilograms per person per year, to 27.7 kg in 2020, with the EU zone as a net importer by 2016.

Europe's prospects for exporting poultry meat during this period are likely to be constrained both by its relatively high production costs and by an assumed strengthening of the Euro currency, so that total exports fall back to below 740,000 metric tons from a 2011 level of about 966,000 tons. By contrast, American analysts have projected that a relative weakness of the U.S., dollar in currency exchange rates will make U.S., exports more competitive.

Within the USA, analysts forecast increased retail prices for meat over the next two years or so, but with added costs of production keeping producer margins tight. They also see the next few years as the time of opportunity for chicken to win U.S., market share against pork and beef by being more available and lower priced. Potentially, domestic chicken production could grow by more than 1.6 per cent over the next decade.

On current assessments, the global demand for eggs could reach 71 million metric tons per year by 2015. The largest increases in egg production between 2011 and 2015 are likely to occur in Brazil, Turkey, India and China. But a longer-term view also points to China and India having the greatest demand for more eggs because of more mouths to feed. By 2050, these two countries are expected to hold a combined one-third of the global human population. Egg forecasts of the percentage growth in production weight, comparing 2015 with 2011, range between only 0.6

per cent in the European Union and 0.3 per cent in Japan, to 9 per cent to 10 per cent in China and Indonesia, 14 per cent in India and Turkey, and 17 per cent in Brazil. Already representing the fastest regional growth rate in egg production since 2000, Asia has also been identified as the driver of further increases in the global average number of eggs consumed per person annually. The current average is about 175 eggs per person, but may exceed 200 within the next 8 to 9 years.

Currently, less than 2 per cent of eggs are traded internationally compared to 60 per cent of beef. However, demand from developing countries is expected to drive the total egg market to a 20 per cent expansion over the next 10 years, bringing with it an increase in the trading of egg products.

ORGANIC PRODUCTION OF POULTRY

Any number of pasture-based systems can be classified as organic if the producer chooses to follow the certification process which requires that feed, pasture and processor be certified organic. In terms of organic production, the USDA'S National Organic Programme requires outdoor access and organic feeds produced without synthetic chemicals and prohibits the use of antibiotics (USDA NOP, 2006; Fanatico, 2007). In Florida, there are a number of producers that follow organic standards for raising their flock but have chosen not to become certified organic for various reasons. The main drawback of organic production is the elevated cost of feed and the lack of processing facilities that offer services for certified organic producers.

Opportunities of Pastured Poultry Production

According to the National Center for Appropriate Technology (NCAT), there is a strong demand for pasture-raised poultry products when marketed directly to consumers. These types of operations can be managed by one person and producers can start small and grow as they become proficient in producing and marketing poultry and/or eggs. There is minimal initial capital investment compared to most agricultural enterprises. However, poultry products can also attract customers for other products. Moreover, pastured poultry production is arguably a more sustainable system because the nutrients in poultry excreta are being deposited into the soil. These deposits serve as a source of organic matter and nutrients that help build soil fertility, assist water retention and increase forage production. This can be especially beneficial in areas with deep sandy soils and low fertility.

Challenges of Pastured Poultry Production

The challenges associated with pasture-raised poultry are labour, seasonality and processing. This is a labour intensive operation: the birds will need to be fed, watered and moved at least once–and sometimes twice–daily. Meat production in North Florida is mostly seasonal with production and harvest ranging from February to June and August to December in order to avoid extremes in temperature. The climactic conditions will dictate how early or late in the season birds can stay in the pasture because weather related stress can affect feed conversion and meat quality. On the other hand, laying flocks can cope with varying climactic conditions if adequate housing is provided. Predation pressure also presents challenges, especially for new producers because it takes time to develop predator control strategies to minimize losses.

Meat Birds: Breed Selection

Unlike with laying hens there are limited breed options for meat birds. The options include the Cornish cross hybrids which are selected for commercial production systems. Cornish crosses are considered a fast-growing broiler. These broilers reach a market weight of five to six pounds in approximately seven to eight weeks. Due to the fact that Cornish cross broilers are harvested at a younger age their meat tends to be more tender and juicy and does not exhibit a strong flavour like heritage birds.

An emerging trend in pastured poultry production is the use of dual purpose heritage breeds to help preserve the genetic pool of poultry in the United States. Heritage breeds are breeds recognised by the American Poultry Association prior to the mid 20th century. Heritage breeds include barred silvers and dual purpose breeds like New Hampshire, Buff Orpington and Barred Rocks. With dual purpose poultry breeds males are selected for meat production and females for egg production. The dual purpose chicken will not provide a large carcass as a meat bird, nor lay as many eggs as an egg layer. These birds tend to grow slowly, eat more feed and may take up to 12 weeks to reach market weight. Heritage breeds are also considered to have a stronger flavour because the age at which the birds are killed and processed is an important factor that contributes to flavour. Breed selection will be based on your preferences and in some instances the preferences of your market and consumer demand.

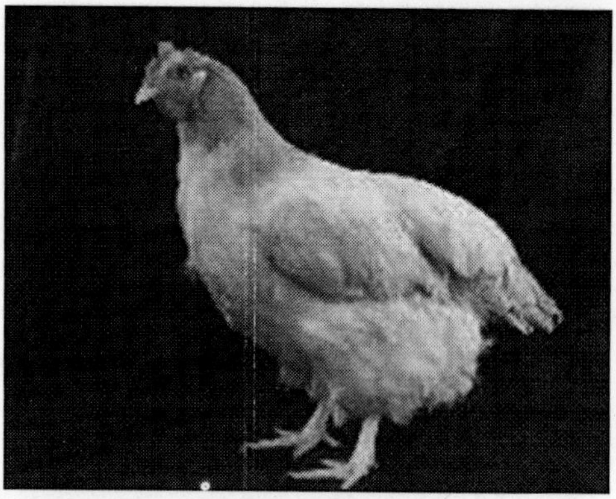

Fig: Buff Orpington Hen.

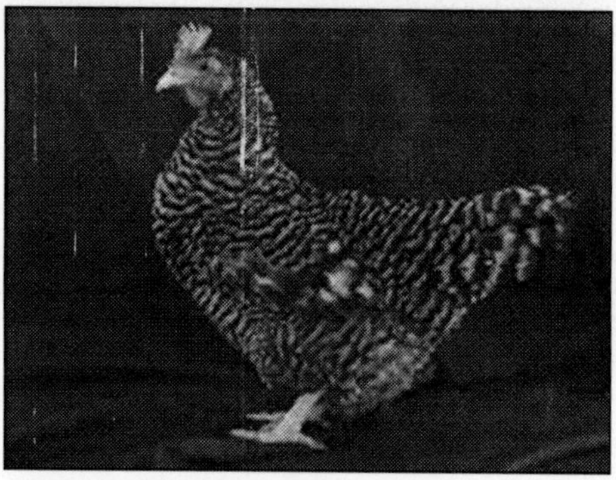

Fig: Barred Rock Hen.

Selecting Laying Hens

Commercial hatcheries offer a wide variety of options when it comes to laying hens. A common misconception is that hybrids are man-made breeds. In reality hybrids are a cross between known breeds whose offspring will usually grow faster, provide flock uniformity and increased egg production. This is often referred to as hybrid vigour. Some examples of hybrids include red sex links, production reds and white leghorns. Once again, personal preference and market will drive the breed selection process.

Heritage breeds are also an option in a layer operation. A benefit of using heritage breeds is the conservation of genetic diversity. Some of the breeds in this category include New Hampshire, Rhode Island Red, Buff Orpington, Minorca and Ancona. Additionally, heritage breeds have adapted to changing environmental conditions and are natural and efficient foragers. Using this type of bird in a pasture-based production system can also be used as a marketing tool.

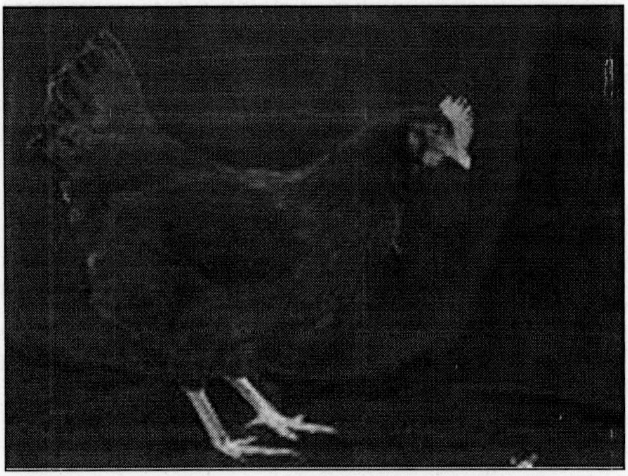

Fig: Rhode Island Red Hen.

Some products prefer to select a breed based on the colour of eggs desired. A rule of thumb for brown and white egg layers is the colour of the bird's ear lobes will, in many cases, correspond to the colour of the eggs which they will lay. White Leghorns are among the most popular and productive layers of white eggs whereas Rhode Island Reds are the second most popular and produce large brown eggs. If more unique shell colour or "designer eggs" are desired then the Araucana and Ameracana breeds will provide these results.

Starting the Birds

In a pasture-based poultry system newly hatched chicks will not go directly into the pasture. During the first couple of weeks an enclosed structure is needed in order to provide temperature regulation, feed and water. This enclosed structure is more commonly known as a brooder. In the case of broilers, the chicks will remain in the brooder for approximately three weeks or until they are sufficiently feathered to withstand climactic conditions. In contrast, chicks that will later become layers will need to remain in the brooder for approximately six weeks. These first couple of weeks will determine the long term survival, development and health of the flock in the pasture.

The brooder should meet the following requirements:

- One-half of a square foot per bird.
- A heat source (infra red lamps are recommended, have two in case one burns out).
- Three inches of dry bedding such as wood shavings, hay or straw. Try to avoid slippery surfaces like newspaper.

- One quart of water for every 25 birds.
- Clean feeders. The feeder should be placed near the heat source, but not directly underneath it.
- Some form of ventilation. Chicks need draft protection, but proper ventilation during the brooding period is very important.

During the first week, the temperature in the brooder should remain a constant 95 degrees Fahrenheit. After the first week the temperature should be lowered five degrees per week for the next two to three weeks, after the third week the birds are typically ready to be moved into the pasture. The temperature in the brooder can be decreased by raising the heat source. It is very important that fresh water and feed be offered ad libitum (free choice) daily because it is vital for their growth and health once they are in the pastures. Care should be taken to insure that the feed and water are not allowed to become too warm because this will result in the chicks not eating and drinking as much as they need.

On delivery day, you need to have the brooder up and running 24 hours before the chicks arrive in order to detect any problems beforehand. Also make sure that the hatchery sends the chicks via overnight mail to avoid losses and to get the chicks to starting drinking and eating feed. When placing the birds in the brooder each bird should be introduced to the water source by dipping their beak directly into the water.

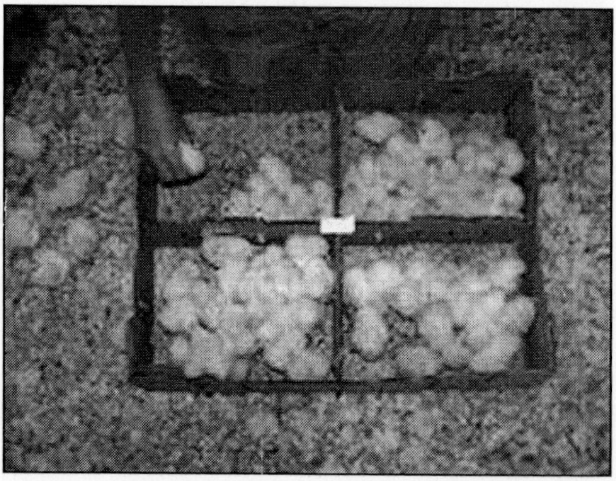

Fig: Baby Chicks on Delivery Day.

U.S., consumers are increasingly interested in products they perceive as naturally-produced or environmentally-friendly, that provide a high level of nutrition, good flavour, improved welfare for the birds, and provide information about how the food was produced. These interests have led to specialty markets for poultry produced in alternative systems such as free-

Ostrich and Emu Production

Ostrich and Emu farming is now-a-days considered to be one of the most profitable agricultural projects. They are referred as 'farms of the future' due to the large variety of products and hence the high profits potential. Ostrich meat is highly nutritive and earns enormous foreign exchange. Ostriches are raised commercially for their egg, meat, feathers and hide. The increased consumer awareness of the problems of cholesterol in the blood and their possible association of heart attacks and arteriosclerosis, the demand for ostrich meat in international market began to increase. A number of beef producers in Europe, America and Canada have most recently switched to commercial ostrich farming due to higher and faster financial returns on ostrich projects. Ostrich meat is in great demand in European and American countries and is already extremely popular and available in most of the restaurants and supermarkets.

Recently Tamil Nadu Veterinary and Animal Sciences University imported 100 chicks from Malaysia. Their adaptability to climatic conditions prevailing in the state would be tested and if successful it will be recommended to the interested farmers and entrepreneurs. Considering the above aspects of alternate poultry production, our country has a great potential to develop further in this area of farm production. The NABARD and associated banks are also ready with model projects and financing of such projects through reimbursement scheme which is also a boost for future developments.

Role in Indian Poultry Production

Remarkable growth of poultry sector in the Indian sub-continent has been essentially chicken dominated; dependent on intensive system of production involving high technology with high external inputs. This is not necessarily appropriate and sustainable to the socio-economy of a densely populated country facing routine shortage of conventional poultry feed resources. The prevailing socio-agro-economic scenario of this sub-continent calls for some kind of cafeteria approach for poultry production; scientists should develop and offer a broad spectrum of poultry alternatives to meet the different local requirements. The availability of such diversification possibilities would maximize the returns from a given level of inputs and also minimize the risks and hazards to the environment. In this context, importance of alternate poultry species is being rediscovered. Production of alternate poultry may never rise enough to compete with commercial chicken, but these birds could become a significant source of food for the masses and also a source for substantial supplement income.

Guinea fowl and turkeys are interesting gallinaceous birds being farmed for centuries to meet poultry production requirements of diversified eco- agriculture mellieu. The traditionally raised guinea fowl and turkey ensure reasonable returns at insignificant cash inputs, while quail production is a distinct diversification offer. Intimate understanding of the basics of domestication; disease control, nutrition and genetics has helped farm production of these avian species. Present paper covers the present and future importance of these alternate poultry germplasm resources available in the country.

Germplasm Resources

Guinea fowl were introduced into the Indian sub-continent during the slavery era of mediaeval centuries. Preliminary survey of guinea fowl showed its distinct popularity with marginal farmers and other vulnerable groups as small-scale poultry enterprise. The indigenous germplasm seems well adapted to the diversified agro-climatic conditions prevailing in semi-arid regions. Guinea fowl population rank third after chickens and ducks. It is referred to by different regional names in this sub-continent 'Titari in northern plains; and 'Chittra' in the Majority of guinea fowl are raised in\ semi-arid pockets of Punjab,Uttar Pradesh, Bihar, Rajasthan, Madhya Pradesh, Maharashtra, Saurashtra, Karnataka, Andhra Pradesh, Orissa and Tamil Nadu. Present production status in this country is best summed up as widely spread and highly fragmented.

The descriptions of guinea fowl breeds/ varieties are essentially based on the plumage colour variations. Pearl, Lavender and White are the three main varieties recognised world over. In India, Pearl guinea fowl are most common among village stocks and usually referred as the 'local' breed. Pearl individuals are characterised by dark-gray feathers with uniformly distributed white spots that present a pearl like appearance. Pearl plumage, colour is also regarded as the 'wild' mutant. Levender birds are identified by their light gray distinctly spotted feathers. White variety possesses completely white plumage. Guncari guinea fowl stocks developed at the Central Avian Research Institute, Izatnagar are selected for high early body weight and breed true to their plumage characteristics. Some minor plumage mutant varieties, viz., Violet, Lilac, White breasted pearl and White breasted lavender also available.

Ecogenetic Potentials

The ecogenetic characterisation is identification of species specific potentials to survive under non-conductive harsh environments. Evolved in tropics, guineafowl is considered to possess relatively higher level of tolerance for rigourous tropical climatic conditions. Although no detailed studies are reported but preliminary observations indicate existence of better potentials.

Body conformation and plumage cover are the two important factors in determination of heat tolerance potentials. Light in body weight, long-legged guinea fowl present greater surface area for heat dissipation per unit body weight. Low feather weight estimates (7.8 per cent) at 12-week to 16-week age are comparatively lower than the average values reported for different domestic fowl classes. Long neck devoid of feathers, poorly feathered thighs, exposed and highly vascular nares, cere, wattles and helmet play important role in thermoregulation. Its more fluffy monotype plumage covering and potential to elevate feathers permit better circulation of air through plumage, more efficient dissipation of internal heat.

Normal respiratory actions and stress panting with outstretched wing help dissipation of internal heat through vaporisation movement. The normal respiratory frequency for guinea fowl is not different from that of chicken (18-30 breaths/min). Experiments revealed comparatively little polypnea during moderately high ambient temperature (85°C - 110°F) among guinea fowl vis- à-vis chicken. Mycotoxin contamination of feed grains is more common in tropical and sub-tropical countries, particularly when coupled with poor handling operations. The higher aflatoxin tolerance of guinea fowl indicates it potential to utilise lower quality feed ingredients.

Production Systems

Guinea fowl may be raised in the modern intensive system characterised by high input, good husbandry and hygiene and supply of balanced feed, however this system is confined largely to Government/ public sector farms. The traditional extensive system of rearing is most popular in rural areas. A limited survey showed that birds are maintained in complete harmony to the village environment; housing and management is completely traditional and birds are raised on free range. Average flock size varies widely (15-200) in guinea fowl producing pockets. Droving is the most popular form of husbandry. Birds offer no management problems, primarily due to their flocking instincts. In semi-extensive system, birds are maintained in pens communicating with spacious well-fenced enclosures. Management is entirely through incorporation of family labour; two persons can easily manage even large flocks. In the traditional rearing system, the nutritional requirements of voraciously omnivorous guinea fowl are met through its catholic feeding habits; birds accept fallen grains, leaves, weeds, root-bulbs, fruits, diversified insect fauna and flora and even carrion. Supplementary feeding, if any, usually consist of waste grains, household waste and crop residues.

Strategies of combining guinea fowl raising with arable crops, fruit plantations and pastures for ruminant production contribute towards the production economy as well as stability of the system.

Its advantages include:

- More complete utilisation of land,
- Control of waste herbage, weed growth and the insect pests,
- Increased land fertility and
- The plantation environment reduces heat stress to birds during foraging activities.

Several reports indicate that guinea fowl may be beneficially integrated with crops of rice, ragi, grapes, apple and ruminant farming, etc., because of its potentials to minimize the harmful insect pests and weeds. Our observations strongly suggest complete economic viability of guinea fowl production. A study of inputs and returns showed reasonable net gains for guinea fowl production when 2-3 crops of at least 500 heats are raised every year on foraging: particularly when mortality was kept under control. In view of the increasing demands for more and more diversity in poultry meat, and elite class consumer preferences for the native free range fed poultry products, there seems and ample scope for the guinea fowl produce.

Germplasm Resources

Although, turkeys were introduced in this subcontinent continent several decades back by the Christian missionaries, but till date turkey farming has achieved very little progress as well popularity. Possibly high cost of production, long generation interval and less market demand are the main reasons for its low popularity.

A study conducted at HAU, Hisar showed that production price of 1 kg live weight of turkey was more than 1.5 times higher that that of broilers. Generally speaking, turkey production has failed to generate popular interest in most of the tropical countries outside Latin America. Recently, it has atso started gaining popularity in several African countries. Bronze, White Holland Bourbon Red, Narangansett, Black, Slate and Beltsville Small White (BSW) are the standard breeds. Among a dozen or more non-standard varieties, Broad Breasted Large White (BBLW) and Broad Breasted Bronze (BBB) are more popular. The white-feathered turkeys are mutants of the original Bronze birds. White birds are preferred over coloured ones because coloured birds contain a black pigment in their quill feathers. In India, Beltsville Small White type turkeys are being maintained at most of the Government/university experimental farms. At few centers, Broad Breasted Bonze and Broad Breasted Large White units are also being kept.

Organised turkey farms under private sector are practically non-existent, limited to few small units at Government/public sector farms. Domestic turkey maintained at private small-scale units scattered throughout the country are mainly the decendents of semi-improved

Broad Breasted Bronze turkey imported from Europe and North America during the early ears and it is referred to as local breed. Few flocks of Norfolks and Cambridge turkeys, may be also there. The total turkey population is small, may be one lakh birds are raised annually. These unimproved turkeys are produced as a cash crop for meeting the market needs for Christmas dinner, birth days, wedding or holidays treats.

Ecogenetic Potentials

Evolved from a truly tropical bird, whose natural habitat was open forests and wooded areas, the present domesticated farms have largely retained its self-reliance, ruggedness and adaptability. They can be reared virtually anywhere.

The hardy 'local' turkey stocks are able to thrive under hot climate to the arid conditions, from sea level to mountains with near temperate climates and from rain forests to deserts. Turkeys walk rather than fly and find almost all their food on ground when kept on range. They possess excellent foraging and scavenging abilities.

Production System

The turkey may be reared under intensive as well as extensive system of rearing. The intensive rearing system is largely restricted to the Government/ public sector.

The intensive management is almost similar to that of chicken and is basically of deep litter type. One sq ft of floor space per poult is required during the first 3-4 weeks and thereafter the floor space requirement per bird is 1.5 sq ft upto 8 th week, 2 sq ft upto 12 th weeks of age, 2.5 sq ft upto 16 th weeks of age and 305 sq ft after 16 th weeks of age.

Free range system of rearing is most popular for rearing the local stocks of turkey. They are natural foragers and scavengers and always range farther. Indeed, they thrive best where they can rove about freely feeding on seeds, fresh grass, other herbage and insects which include locusts, cicadas, crickets; grasshoppers, worms, slugs and snails, etc. The self reliant 'local' stocks cat do well with little management and can still fly short distances to avoid predators.

PRESERVATION OF EGGS

The following precautions are suggested by G. H. Lamson, Jr., of Connecticut: Keep the whole flock of hens in as perfect a state of health as possible. Give enough shell-forming food to form strong shells of uniform thickness. Make proper nesting places and keep nests clean, so eggs may not be infected while in the nests. Gather the eggs each day and keep them in a cool, dry room or cellar where the sun's rays do not fall directly upon them. Use only clean eggs and place them in the preservative within 24 hours after they are laid. Preserve only April, May and early June eggs.

As to methods of preserving undoubtedly cold storage at a temperature of 34 degrees is the best and practically the only method used commercially. But it is too expensive to be practiced on a small scale. Formerly dry methods such as packing in grain or salt were used, but these are no longer recommended, as the eggs lose much of their moisture by evaporation.

Among the liquid preservatives, water glass has been very generally and successfully used because it is reliable, easily prepared and comparatively cheap. Water glass can be bought at most drug stores for $1 or $1.25 a gallon. A gallon will make 10 gallons of preserving fluid. Eggs have been kept in this mixture for three or four years without developing an unpleasant taste or smell, but when kept any longer the yolk becomes pink and very liquid. The white coagulates in the usual manner in cooking.

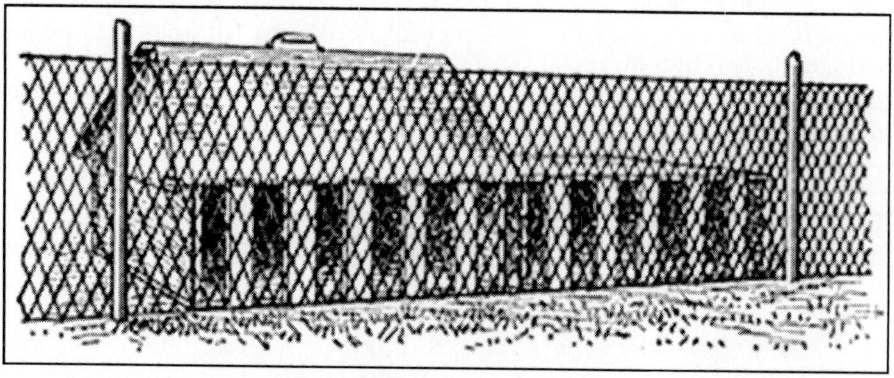

Fig: Fence Protects Coops at Night.

To preserve eggs by this method, a cellar should be used where the temperature does not go above 60 degrees. Any clean water-tight receptacle will do; kegs or stone jars are commonly used. Each receptacle should be scalded thoroughly two or three times to make sure that it is perfectly clean. The preserving fluid should be made from water that has been boiled and allowed to cool. This is mixed at the rate of nine parts water to one of water glass, and thoroughly stirred. The quantity needed for each receptacle should be mixed in that receptacle so as to insure the proper strength of solution. When mixed in one and then poured into several others there is a likelihood of getting different strengths. It is desirable to label each crock or keg with the date the eggs are put down. When filled the receptacle should be kept out of the sun's rays and covered with loose boards. Water should be added from time to time to supply the loss by evaporation and to keep the eggs always beneath the surface. The preservative never should be stirred. When desired for use, the June eggs should be taken first, May eggs next, and April eggs last, because their keeping qualities are different. If eggs are to be sold they should be washed.

One man who has practiced preserving on an extensive scale found that the eggs cost 15 cents a dozen to produce as an average. His market price was 18 cents during spring. The margin of 3 cents profit did not appeal to him, so when eggs came down to 18 cents in March he began preserving. He used only the eggs produced by his own flock. By Thanksgiving time when eggs are selling at 50 and 60 cents a dozen in Boston, he sold these eggs as "storage extras" at an average of 32 cents a dozen, some as high as 40 cents. As the eggs were all produced by his own hens, he could guarantee the quality. This is very important.

The cost of storing was about $2 for 200 dozen. Had these eggs been sold in March at 18 cents they would have brought only $36. By preserving they brought $64, or an apparent net gain of $28. There is, however, another way to look at this which is even more startling. As the average cost to make the eggs was 15 cents, at 18 cents there would have been only 3 cents a dozen profit, or only $6 on the 200 dozen.

By holding until prices were high he actually made 17 cents a dozen instead of 3 cents, or a total profit of $34. It would not be advisable to preserve eggs on a large scale at first. There is a good deal to be learned before one can venture upon this business. The family supply will be enough to lay down as an experiment. After a year or two of experience and confidence will be soon enough to start preserving for the market.

New York State Experiments

At the New York experiment station a number of methods that could be used with little expense on a small scale for preserving eggs, and also some modifications of these methods, show that no method of dry packing gives satisfactory results whether the eggs are turned regularly or not. The best results were secured by keeping the eggs immersed in solutions either of lime, lime and salt, water glass, from 10 to 20 per cent solution, or a proprietary solution consisting largely of water glass.

On the whole, preference is given to a solution of lime and salt to which a little boracic acid was added of a specific gravity somewhat lower than that of eggs. The common materials can be cheaply obtained in pure condition, and the preserved eggs were easier to clean than those from more costly solutions which gave no better results. Though, of course, no preserved egg could grade with a fresh one, little difference in quality of eggs, as tested by many individuals, could be detected between those preserved in the few efficient solutions.

Egg Gathering

Clean eggs always sell at higher prices than soiled ones. In order to secure them, eggs should be gathered at least twice a day, and oftener when the ground is muddy. This applies especially to the summer weather. Eggs quickly begin to decompose when the temperature is high and should, therefore, be removed as soon as possible to a cool dark place.

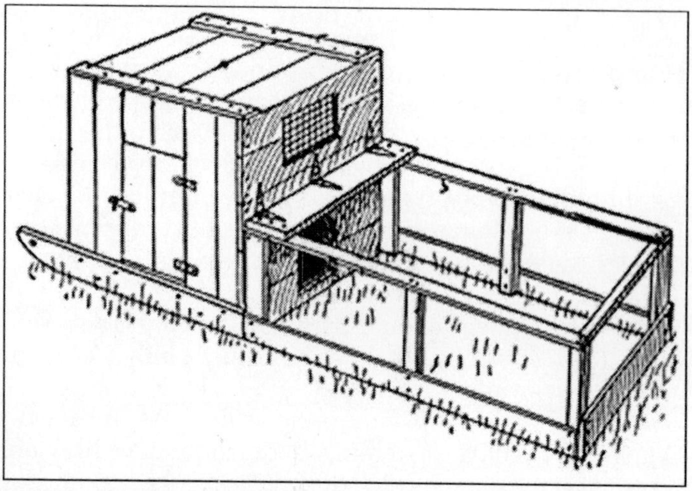

Fig: Portable Coop and Run. Packing Case Coop and Wire Fence Covered Run.

Fertile eggs begin to deteriorate sooner than sterile ones; hence, unless needed for hatching, hens and pullets should be kept by themselves. Fertile eggs, even when fresh laid, may be considered as already started in development. For this reason it is highly desirable that the eggs be gathered frequently, because the warmth of the bodies of several hens on the nest will hasten development of the embryo, and if eggs are allowed to stay in the nest for several hours under such conditions they cannot be considered as strictly fresh.

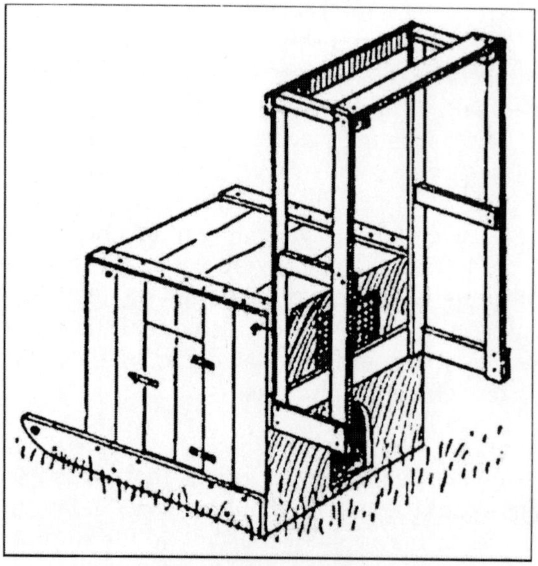

Fig: Ready for Moving.

Until marketed, the clean, fresh eggs, frequently gathered, should be kept in a cool place. Even though this place is clean and cool and it is not dry, the eggs are likely to be injured by mold.

If they become damp and then happen to touch coloured material they are likely to become stained. The best way of holding is to store the eggs in good egg cases in a cool, dry place above the floor. Prior to marketing, the eggs should be graded.

All small, dirty, stained eggs as well as those which have been in the incubator or which are doubtful or rotten should be removed. The small and dirty ones, if fresh, are just as good as the large, clean ones, but they will not sell as well, and if sent to market will injure the price which would be paid for large eggs.

Large eggs, among which small ones are mixed, will sell for the price of the small ones and the buyer, after grading, will sell the large ones at advanced prices and the small ones for what he paid, or better. Therefore, small and soiled eggs should be used at home. Never should eggs be washed, because washing injures the keeping qualities. Every egg from a stolen nest, unless its freshness is unquestionable, should either be thrown away or used at home. The man who wishes to build up a trade cannot afford to risk his chances by letting any such eggs go to market. Eggs handled as suggested should be marketed two or three times a week, oftener if convenient. When so many trips cannot be made, it is well to co-operate with some neighbour to go on alternate days. In autumn and spring, eggs should be marketed not less frequently than once a week.

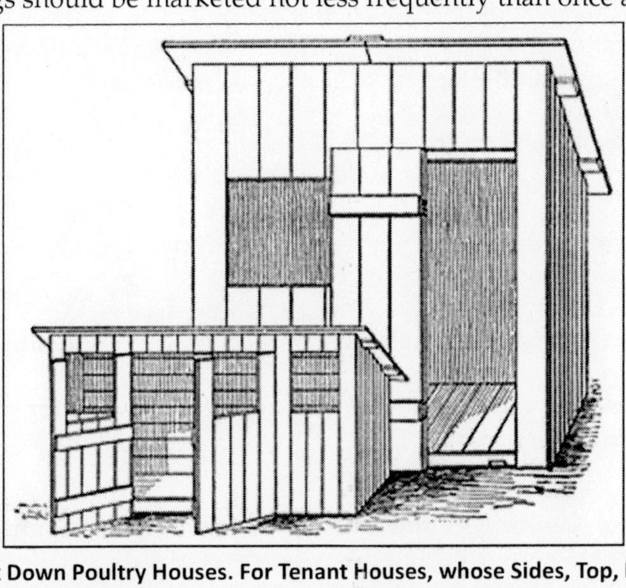

Fig: Knock Down Poultry Houses. For Tenant Houses, whose Sides, Top, Floors and Roofs Bolt Together are Convenient for Moving from Farm to Farm.

It is bad policy to hold eggs in the hope of advancing prices. Evaporation always takes place and the chances are that the grade and the price will be lower than if the eggs are marketed at once; besides, the man who gets the reputation of marketing frequently will always command the respect of his buyers. In hot weather the cases should always be covered to protect them from the heat.

PRESSURE CANNING POULTRY

Follow step-by-step directions for your pressure canner. Process poultry according to the following recipes.

Cut-Up Poultry

Boil, steam, or bake poultry slowly to medium done. I tend to boil it and make the broth at the same time. If you have broth on hand you can precook in the concentrated broth for more flavour. Poultry is medium done when the pink colour in the center is almost gone.

Cut poultry into serving size pieces and if desired, remove bones. I always debone the meat as it is my personal preference. I find it easier to use in recipes if it is done this way. Pack hot poultry loosely in clean, hot Mason jars, leaving 1 1/4-inch head-space.

Make broth from bones and bony pieces, neck, back, and wing tips and the gizzard, heart and liver if you have them. Pack hot meat in clean, hot Mason jars, leaving 1-inch head-space. Do not pack food tightly. Cover poultry with boiling broth or water, leaving 1 1/4-inch head-space. Adjust jar lids.

Poultry may be processed with or without salt. If salt is desired, use only pure canning or pickling salt. Table salt contains a filler which may cause cloudiness in bottom of jar. I use 1/2 teaspoon salt to each pint, 1 teaspoon to each quart.

Dial Gauge Canner: Process at 11 pounds pressure. With Bone: Pints 65 minutes and Quarts 75 minutes. Without Bone: Pints 75 minutes and Quarts 90 minutes.

For processing above 2,000 feet altitude, see above chart for recommended pounds of pressure.

Weighted Gauge Canner: Process at 10 pounds pressure. With Bone: Pints 65 minutes and Quarts for 75 minutes. Without Bone: Pints 75 minutes and Quarts for 90 minutes.

For processing above 1,000 feet altitude, see above chart for recommended pounds of pressure.

Rabbit

Pressure Canning is the Only Safe Method for Canning Rabbit: Follow step-by-step directions for your pressure canner. Process rabbit according to the following recipes.

Soak dressed rabbits 1 hour in water containing 1 tablespoon of salt per quart. Rinse and remove excess fat. Cut into serving size pieces. Boil, steam, or bake to medium done. Rabbit is medium done when pink colour in center is almost gone. Pack hot rabbit loosely in clean, hot Mason jars, leaving 1 1/4- inch head-space. Cover rabbit with boiling broth or water leaving 1 1/4-inch head-space and adjust jar lids.

Dial Gauge Canner: Process at 11 pounds pressure.

With Bone: Pints 65 minutes and Quarts for 75 minutes.

Without Bone: Pints 75 minutes and Quarts for 90 minutes.

For processing above 2,000 feet altitude, see chart for recommended pounds of pressure.

Weighted Gauge Canner:Process at 10 pounds pressure. With Bone: Pints 65 minutes and Quarts for 75 minutes. Without Bone: Pints 75 minutes and Quarts for 90 minutes.

For processing above 1,000 feet altitude, see chart for recommended pounds of pressure.

Altitude chart for canning meat and poultry

Altitude	Dial Gauge Canner Pints and Quarts	Weighted Gauge Canner
Pints and Quarts		
1,001 - 2,000 ft.	11 lbs.	15 lbs.
2,001 - 4,000 ft.	12 lbs.	15 lbs.
4,001 - 6,000 ft.	13 lbs.	15 lbs.
6,001 - 8,000 ft.	14 lbs.	15 lbs.

□

4

Types of Poultry Diseases

AMYLOIDOSIS

A Coronavirus infection of chickens with a morbidity of 50-100 per cent and a mortality 0-25 per cent, depending on secondary infections. Infection is via the conjunctiva or upper respiratory tract with an incubation period of 18-36 hours. The infection spreads rapidly by contact, fomites or aerosol. Some birds/viral strains can be carriers for up to 1 year. The virus, which may survive 4 weeks in premises, is sensitive to solvents, heat (56°C for 15 mins), alkalis, disinfectants (Formal 1 per cent for 3 mins). Poor ventilation and high density are predisposing factors.

Signs

- Sudden death.
- Muscular shivering.
- Otherwise as for standard IB.

Post-mortem Lesions

- Oedema of pectoral muscles and subcutaneously on abdomen, lesions progress to necrosis and scarring of deep pectorals in convalescence.
- In layers the ovules may be intensely congested.
- Other lesions of 'classical' IB may be encountered.

Diagnosis

3-5 passages in CE allantoic cavity, HA-, typical lesions, FA, ciliostatic in tracheal organ culture, cell culture (Vero, CK) only after adaptation Serology: HI, Elisa (both group specific), SN (type specific), DID (poor sensitivity, short duration, group specific).

Treatment

Sodium salicylate 1gm/litre (acute phase) where permitted - antibiotics to control secondary colibacillosis (q.v.).

Prevention

Live vaccines of appropriate sero-type and attenuation, possible reactions depending on virulence and particle size.

ARIZONA INFECTION, ARIZONOSIS

Caused by the bacterium Arizona hinshawii, renamed Salmonella Arizonae. It affects turkeys, mainly in North America, and is not present in the UK turkey population.

Mortality is 10-50 per cent in young birds, older birds are asymptomatic carriers. Transmission is vertical, transovarian, and also horizontal, through faecal contamination of environment, feed etc, from long-term intestinal carriers, rodents, reptiles.

Signs

- Dejection.
- Inappetance.
- Diarrhoea.
- Vent-pasting.
- Nervous signs.
- Paralysis.
- Blindness, cloudiness in eye.
- Huddling near heat.

Post-mortem Lesions

- Enlarged mottled liver.
- Unabsorbed yolk sac.
- Congestion of duodenum.
- Cheesy plugs in intestine or caecum.
- Foci in lungs.
- Salpingitis.
- Ophthalmitis.
- Pericarditis.
- Perihepatitis.

Diagnosis

Isolation and identification, methods as per Salmonella spp. Differentiate from salmonellosis, coli-septicaemia.

Treatment

Injection of streptomycin, spectinomycin, or gentamycin at the hatchery is used in some countries. Formerly in-feed medication with nitrofurans was also used.

Prevention

Eradicate from breeder population, fumigation of hatching eggs, good nest and hatchery hygiene, inject eggs or poults with antibiotics, monitor sensitivity.

ASPERGILLOSIS

A fungal infectious disease, caused by Aspergillus fumigatus, in which the typical sign is gasping for breath, especially in young chicks. Sometimes the same organism causes eye lesions or chronic lesions in older birds. The fungus can infect plant material and many species of animals including birds and man. Occasionally similar lesions are produced by other species of Aspergillus or even other fungi such as Penicillium, Absidia etc.

It affects chickens, turkeys, ducks, penguins, game birds, waterfowl, etc, worldwide. The infection has an incubation period of 2-5 days. Morbidity is usually low, but may be as high as 12 per cent. Mortality among young affected birds is 5-50 per cent. Transmission is by inhalation exposure to an environment with a high spore count; there is usually little bird-to-bird transmission. Spores are highly resistant to disinfectants.

Signs

- Acute form:
- Inappetance.
- Weakness.
- Silent gasping.
- Rapid breathing.
- Thirst.
- Drowsiness.
- Nervous signs (rare).
- Chronic Forms:
- Ocular discharge (ocular form only).
- Wasting.

Post-mortem Lesions

- Yellow to grey nodules or plaques in lungs, air sacs, trachea, plaques in peritoneal cavity, may have greenish surface.
- Conjunctivitis/keratitis.
- Brain lesions may be seen in some birds with nervous signs.

Diagnosis

This is usually based on the signs and lesions and microscopic examination for the fungus, preferably after digestion in 10 per cent potassium hydroxide. It may be confirmed by isolation of the fungus, typically by putting small pieces of affected tissue on Sabouraud agar. Growth occurs in 24-48 hours and colonies are powdery green/blue in appearance. Differentiate from excessive exposure to formalin or vaccinal reactions in day olds and from heat stress in older birds.

Treatment

Usually none. Environmental spraying with effective antifungal antiseptic may help reduce challenge. Amphotericin B and Nystatin have been used in high-value birds.

Prevention

Dry, good quality litter and feed, hygiene, Thiabendazole or Nystatin has been used in feed.

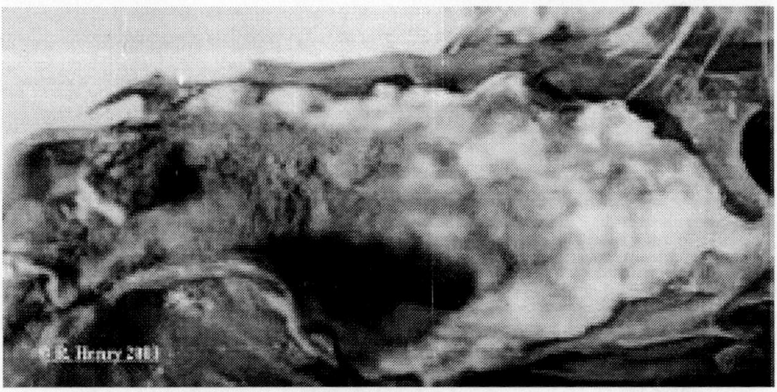

Fig: 'Furry' Airsacculitis in Aspergillosis of an Adult Duck. The Powdery Surface is Dark Green in Colour.

AVIAN ENCEPHALOMYELITIS EGG DROP

Avian encephalomyelitis virus infection in laying bird causes inapparent infection or drops in egg production. It affects chickens, turkeys, quail, pheasants and occurs in most poultry-producing countries. Morbidity 5-60 per cent, mortality none. The means of transmission is unknown but probably by faecal contamination of environment, feed, water etc. with an oral infection route. Virus in faeces may survive 4 weeks or more. Predisposed by immunosuppression.

Signs

- Drop in egg production, small (5-10 per cent) and lasting no more than 2 weeks. and there is serious disease in the progeny.

Post-mortem Lesions

- None.

Diagnosis

History, rising titre to AE virus, subsequent disease in progeny if breeders. Serology - The embryo protection test has been used in the past, now Elisa is used more commonly. Differentiate from Infectious Bronchitis, lentogenic Newcastle disease, EDS-76.

Treatment

None.

Prevention

Vaccination of breeders/layers at 9-15 weeks, attenuated or not. Immunity is usually long lasting.

AVIAN LEUKOSIS, LYMPHOID LEUKOSIS, LEUKOSIS/SARKOMA GROUP

A complex of viral diseases with various manifestations such as lymphoid leukosis, myeloblastosis, erythroblastosis, osteopetrosis, myxosarcomas, fibrosarcomas, other tumours. It affects chickens worldwide with susceptibility varying considerably among different strains and types of stock - egg layers are generally more susceptible to lymphoid leukosis.

Morbidity is low but mortality high. Mortality tends to be chronically higher than normal for a prolonged period. Egg production is somewhat reduced. There may be increased susceptibility to other infectious diseases due to damage to the immune system. Vertical transmission is most important by infection of the egg white in infected breeders (who are long-term carriers), lateral transmission is poor but infection may occur by the faecal-oral route, especially in young birds. In lymphoid leukosis the incubation period is about 4-6 months; it may be as short as 6 weeks for some of the other manifestations. The causative viruses are rapidly inactivated at ambient temperature and on exposure to most disinfectants.

Signs

- Depression.
- Emaciation.
- Loss of weight.
- Persistent low mortality.
- Enlargement of abdomen, liver or bursa.
- Many are asymptomatic.

Post-mortem Lesions

- Focal grey to white tumours, initially in the bursa, then liver, spleen, kidney etc. Liver may be very large.
- Microscopic - cells lymphoplastic

Diagnosis

History, age, lesions, cytology. Differentiate from Marek's disease, coligranuloma.

Treatment

None.

Prevention

Good hygiene, all-in/all-out production, control arthropods, eradication - checking of antigen in the albumen is a basis for eradication.

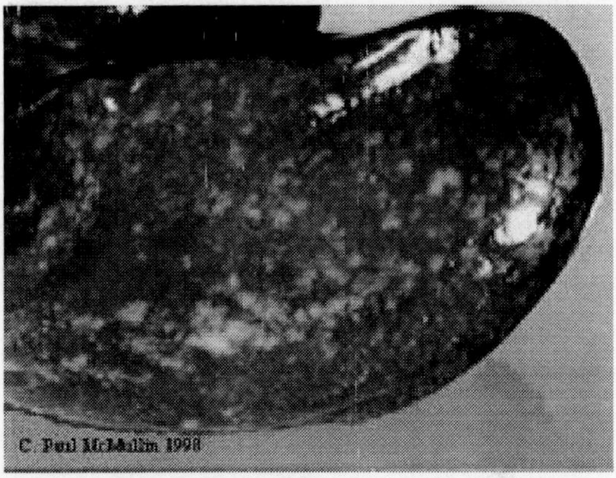

Fig: Diffuse Lymphoid Tumours in an Enlarged Liver from a Mature Broiler Parent Hen.

BIG LIVER AND SPLEEN DISEASE

This condition was first seen in Australia in 1980. It is now known to be caused by an Avian Hepevirus. Related viruses have been reported to cause a hepatitis/splenomegaly syndrome in the USA, sub-clinical infection in pigs and Type E Hepatitis in man. The pig origin virus can cause disease in man, but avian hepeviruses are believed not to be zoonotic. The lesions are associated with deposition of antigen/antibody complexes in tissues. Only chickens are known to be naturally affected, most commonly broiler parents in lay. Natural though it is possible that vertical transmission and/or infection in rear occurs with a subsequent period of latency. Transmission is usually by the faecal/ oral route. Faecal contamination of drinking water is likely to be an efficient means of spread of this infection. Embryos inoculated intravenously become persistently antigen positive.

Signs

- Chronic under production or egg drops of up to 20 per cent.
- Mortality of up to 1 per cent per week for 3-4 weeks.
- Anaemia.
- Premature moulting.

Post-mortem Lesions

- Enlarged spleen (over 1gm/kg bodyweight, often with pale foci).
- Liver usually enlarged, sometimes with subcapsular haemorrhage.

Affected birds may also have:

- Lung congestion
- Ovarian regression
- Yolk peritonitis
- Pale foci and haemorrhages in pancreas.

Diagnosis

Typical signs and lesions. Must be confirmed by laboratory tests. Serological tests (agar gel immunodiffusion) may be used to detect either the specific antigen (which is likely to be positive first) or the antibody response to it. Elisa tests have been developed experimentally. A RT-PCR test may be used to detect viral RNA in tissues. Viral particles may be demonstrated in bile. Histopathology may also be used but the findings are not specific to this condition.

Treatment

No specific treatment known. It may be helpful to control other conditions which may be occurring at the same time. Drinking water which is well chlorinated should be helpful in reducing challenge by this route.

Prevention

Thorough cleaning and disinfection after depletion of an affected flock. Good biosecurity. All-in/all-out production.

BOTULISM

A condition of chickens, turkeys, ducks and other waterfowl occurring worldwide and caused by a bacterial toxin produced by Clostridium botulinum mainly types A/ C. The toxin is produced in decaying animal (usually carcases) and plant waste, and toxin-containing material (pond-mud, carcases, maggots) is consumed by the birds. Toxin may also be produced by the bacteria in the caecum. Morbidity is usually low but mortality is high. The toxin and bacterial spores are relatively stable and may survive for some time in the environment. It has also been suggested that poultry carcases lost in litter can be a cause of botulism in cattle grazing land or consuming silage where poultry litter has been spread.

Signs

- Nervous signs, weakness, progressive flaccid paralysis of legs, wings then neck, then sudden death.
- Affected broilers tend to settle with eyes closed when not disturbed.
- A soiled beak, because it rests on the litter, is also quite typical.

Post-mortem Lesions

- Possibly no significant lesions.
- Mild enteritis if has been affected for some time.
- Feathers may be easily pulled (chicken only).
- Maggots or putrid ingesta may be found in the crop.

Diagnosis

History, signs, mouse toxicology on serum or extract of intestinal contents. Differentiate from acute Marek's disease ('Floppy Broiler Syndrome') by histology of the brain.

Treatment

Remove source of toxin, supportive treatment if justifiable, antibiotics, selenium.

Prevention

Preventing access to toxin, suspect food and stagnant ponds, especially in hot weather. The single most important measure is careful pick-up and removal of all dead birds on a daily basis. This will reduce the risk of botulism both in the poultry and in any grazing animals on land where poultry litter is spread.

CAMPYLOBACTER INFECTION

Campylobacter spp. are bacteria that commonly infect a broad range of livestock species, pets and wild animals. In poultry they tend to multiply in large numbers in the hindgut, principally in the caecae. Campylobacters are a significant cause of enteritis in man. Infected poultry are a potential reservoir of this zoonosis.

Campylobacter jejuni is the commonest species found in poultry. All campylobacters are delicate organisms that survive for relatively short periods outside the host unless protected by organic material, biofilm or engulfed by protozoa.

Campylobacter jejuni infection is not currently considered to be pathogenic in poultry though a Campylobacter-like organism is considered to be the cause of 'Vibrionic Hepatitis'.

There are indications that plantar pododermatitis, carcase quality and litter quality are better on farms which tend to have Campylobacter-negative stock. The reason for this is unclear. It may be that management that favours dry litter reduces the risk of infection and/or transmission within the flock. There is an annual cycle with increased risk of infection in the summer months in some countries.

Diagnosis

Isolation of the organism from caecal contents, cloacal swabs or composite faeces. The organism is sensitive to air so swabs should be collected into transport medium and other samples placed in airtight containers with minimal airspace. Samples should be tested as quickly as possible after collection.

Treatment

Not required on clinical grounds.

Prevention

In principle, housed poultry can be maintained free of Campylobacter infection by consistent application of excellent biosecurity. Key aspects of this include effective sanitation of drinking water, sourcing of water from high quality supplies, avoidance of contact with pets and other farmed species, good hand hygiene by stockmen, and changing of overalls and boots on entering bird areas. In practice the success of this will also depend upon the degree of environmental contamination by the organism. For this reason it may be difficult to stop the spread of infection between houses once it becomes established in one house.

Many infections are introduced during thinning or other forms of partial depopulation. Insects and rodents may act as a means of transfer of the infection from the general environment into the poultry buildings. Research is ongoing on the development of vaccines, phage treatments and competitive exclusion approaches, as well as processing plant technologies to reduce carcase contamination.

CHLAMYDIOSIS, PSITTACOSIS, ORNITHOSIS

An infection of turkeys, ducks, psittacines, pigeons, man, rarely chickens, caused by Chlamydia psittaci, a bacterium of highly variable pathogenicity. It is a 'Scheduled Disease' rarely diagnosed in UK, but occurring probably worldwide.

Morbidity is 50-80 per cent, mortality 5-40 per cent. It is transmitted by contact, faecal dust and wild bird carriers, especially pigeons and robins. Egg transmission does not occur.

Elementary bodies are highly resistant and can survive in dried faeces for many months. Iodophores and formaldehyde are effective disinfecting agents, phenolics are less so. Intercurrent salmonellosis and, perhaps, other infections may be predisposing factors.

Signs

- Respiratory signs.
- Greenish-yellow diarrhoea.
- Depression.
- Weakness.
- Inappetance.
- Weight loss.
- Nasal discharge.
- Conjunctivitis.
- Occasional transient ataxia in pigeons.
- Production drops in naive laying flocks.

Post-mortem Lesions

- Vascular congestion.
- Wasting.
- Fibrinous pericarditis.
- Airsacculitis.
- Perihepatitis.
- Spleen enlarged and congested, may rupture in pigeons.
- Necrotic foci in liver.
- Fibrinous pneumonia.
- Congested lungs and air sacs in the turkey.

Diagnosis

History, signs, lesions. Intracytoplasmic inclusions are helpful but confirmation requires demonstration of causal organisms (Giemsa stain, IFA).

Serology: complement fixation, Elisa and gel diffusion. Differentiate from Duck viral hepatitis, Duck septicaemia.

Treatment

Tetracycline (200-800 ppm in feed for 3-4 weeks) and/or quinolone medication and supervised slaughter.

Prevention

Biosecurity, exclusion of wild birds.

Live and inactivated vaccines are protective although the former result in carriers and the latter require several applications.

COCCIDIOSIS, ILEORECTAL, E BRUNETTI

A relatively rare form of coccidiosis affecting chickens worldwide caused by Eimeria brunetti.

Of moderate to high pathogenicity, it is found in the terminal ileum, caecum and rectum. Morbidity and mortality are variable.

Signs

- Depression.
- Ruffled feathers.
- Closed eyes.
- Inappetance.
- Poor production.
- Diarrhoea, blood in faeces.

Post-mortem Lesions

- Petechiae and thickening of the distal third or more of intestine, extending into caecal tonsils.
- Severe necrotising enteritis.
- Oocysts in caecum and rectum.

Diagnosis

Signs, lesions, microscopic examination of scrapings. Differentiate from ulcerative enteritis, caecal coccidiosis.

Treatment

Toltrazuril, Sulphonamides, Amprolium, Vitamins A and K in feed or water.

Prevention

Coccidiostats in feed, vaccination by controlled exposure, hygiene. This species is not usually included in vaccines for broilers. There is good immunity to the same parasite in recovered birds.

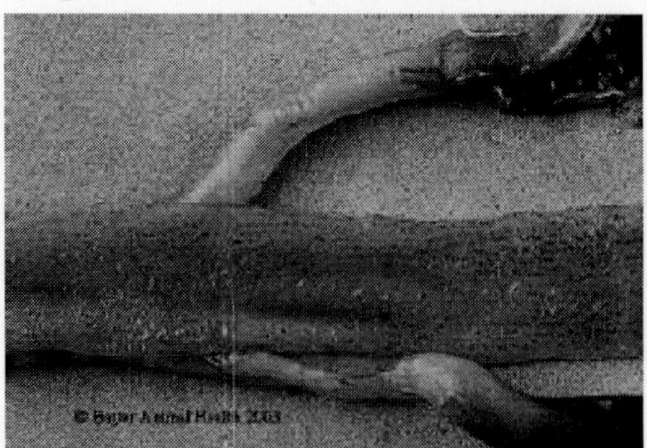

Fig: Moderate Eimeria brunetti Infection in the Terminal Ileum and Rectum of Chicken. There is Thickening of the Intestinal Mucosa and there are Lines of Haemorrhagic Spots in the Mucosa.

COLIBACILLOSIS, COLISEPTICEMIA

Coli-septicaemia is the commonest infectious disease of farmed poultry. It is most commonly seen following upper respiratory disease (such as Infectious Bronchitis) or Mycoplasmosis. It is frequently associated with immunosuppressive diseases such as Infectious Bursal Disease Virus (Gumboro Disease) in chickens or Haemorrhagic Enteritis in turkeys, or in young birds that are immunologically immature. It is caused by the bacterium Escherichia coli and is seen worldwide in chickens, turkeys, etc.

Morbidity varies, mortality is 5-20 per cent. The infectious agent is moderately resistant in the environment, but is susceptible to disinfectants and to temperatures of 80°C. Infection is by the oral or inhalation routes, and via shell membranes/yolk/navel, water, fomites, with an incubation period of 3-5 days. Poor navel healing, mucosal damage due to viral infections and immunosuppression are predisposing factors.

Signs

- Respiratory signs, coughing, sneezing.
- Snick.
- Dejection.
- Reduced appetite.
- Poor growth.
- Omphalitis.

Post-mortem Lesions

- Airsacculitis.
- Pericarditis.
- Perihepatitis.
- Swollen liver and spleen.
- Peritonitis.
- Salpingitis.
- Omphalitis.
- Synovitis.
- Arthritis.
- Enteritis.
- Granulomata in liver and spleen.
- Cellulitis over the abdomen or in the leg.
- Lesions vary from acute to chronic in the various forms of the disease.

Diagnosis

Isolation, sero-typing, pathology. Aerobic culture yields colonies of 2-5mm on both blood and McConkey agar after 18 hours - most strains are rapidly lactose-fermenting producing brick-red colonies on McConkey agar.

Differentiate from acute and chronic infections with Salmonella spp, other enterobacteria such as Proteus, as well as Pseudomonas, Staphylococcus spp. etc.

Treatment

Amoxycillin, tetracyclines, neo-mycin (intestinal activity only), gentamycin or ceftiofur (where hatchery borne), potentiated sulphonamide, flouroquinolones.

Prevention

Good hygiene in handling of hatching eggs, hatchery hygiene, good sanitation of house, feed and water. Well-nourished embryo and optimal incubation to maximise day-old viability. Control of predisposing factors and infections (usually by vaccination). Immunity is not well documented though both autogenous and commercial vaccines have been used.

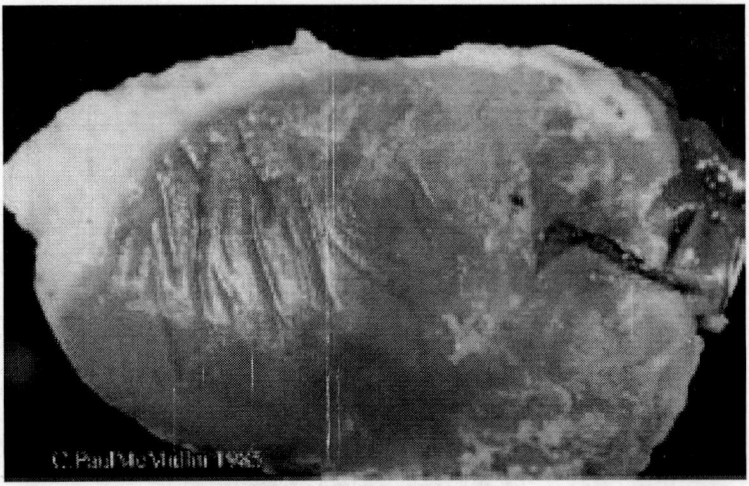

Fig: Severe Perihepatitis in Colibacillosis in a Broiler Parent Chicken.

DEGENERATIVE JOINT DISEASE

A condition of chickens and turkeys seen worldwide. The cause remains to be confirmed, but it may result from physical damage, or developmental defects. Morbidity and mortality are low but affected birds are more likely to be 'picked upon' and may end up suffering damage and needing to be culled. Rapid growth is a possible predisposing factor.

Signs

- Lameness.
- Reduced breeding performance.

Post-mortem Lesions

- Damaged epiphyseal articular cartilage, especially of femoral anti- trochanter but also other leg joints, resulting in erosions, and cartilage flaps.
- Microscopically there is necrosis and there may be fissures of articular cartilage and associated osteochondritis.

Diagnosis

Gross and microscopic lesions.

Treatment

None available. Appropriate management of a segregation pen and early marketing of mildly affected birds may limit losses and improve flock welfare.

Prevention

Avoidance of physical sources of injury to bones and joints. There may be a place for growth-control programmes, especially during period of rapid growth.

ERYSIPELAS

A sudden onset infection with the bacterium Erysipelothrix insidiosa (E. rhusiopathiae) seen in turkeys and increasingly in free-range chickens, rarely in geese, ducks, pheasants. It is also seen in some mammals. It may be transmitted by faecal carriers for 41 days, in soil, water, fishmeal and semen and by cannibalism. The bacterium is fairly resistant to environmental effects or disinfectants and may persist in alkaline soil for years. There is likely to be an increased risk if housing or land has been previously used by pigs or sheep.

Signs

- Inappetance.
- Depression.
- Sleepiness.
- Swollen snood.
- May be diarrhoea and respiratory signs.
- Perineal congestion.
- Chronic scabby skin, especially snood.
- Sudden death.

Post-mortem Lesions

- Carcase congestion.
- Liver, kidney, spleen swollen.
- Haemorrhages in fat, muscle, epicardium.
- Marked catarrhal enteritis.
- Joint lesions.
- Endocarditis.

Diagnosis

Isolation on blood agar, and identification; the demonstration of the organism in stained impression smears from tissues. Vaccination or natural infection may cause false positive reactions in the Mycoplasma gallisepticum and M. synoviae plate tests for a few weeks. Differentiate from pasteurellosis, salmonellosis, colibacillosis, and acute Newcastle disease.

Treatment

Penicillin - a combination of the procaine and benzathine salts may be injected, often along with bacterin. Tetracyclines in feed may also be helpful.

Prevention

Good biosecurity to prevent spread from other susceptible species, vaccine at 16-20 weeks if the condition is enzootic.

GAPE

Syngamus trachea, a nematode worm parasite of chickens, turkeys, pheasants, and other game and ornamental birds occurring worldwide. Infection is by the oral route with earthworms, slugs and snails acting as transfer hosts but the life cycle may also be direct, by ingestion of embryonated egg or L3. There is an 18-20 day prepatent period. The condition is seen more commonly in poultry on free range where ground may be contaminated by wild birds e.g. from rookeries.

Signs

- Gaping.
- Dyspnoea.
- Head shaking.
- Loss of appetite and condition.

Post-mortem Lesions

- Tracheitis.
- Presence of worms, paired parasites up to 2 cm long.

Diagnosis

Signs and lesions, confirmation of presence of the parasite.

Treatment

Flubendazole in feed, levamisole.

Prevention

Flubendazole.

INFECTIOUS BRONCHITIS, IB EGG-LAYERS

A Coronavirus infection of chickens, with much antigenic variation. The condition has a morbidity of 10-100 per cent and mortality of 0-1 per cent. Infection is via the conjunctiva or upper respiratory tract. There is rapid spread by contact, fomites or aerosol.

A few birds are carriers up to 49 days post infection. The virus is moderately resistant and may survive 4 weeks in premises. Poor ventilation and high density are predisposing factors.

Signs

- Drop in egg production (20-50 per cent).
- Soft-shelled eggs.
- Rough shells.
- Loss of internal egg quality.
- Coughing, sneezing.
- Rales may or may not be present.

Post-mortem Lesions

- Follicles flaccid.
- Yolk in peritoneal cavity (non-specific).

Diagnosis

3-5 passages in CE, HA-, typical lesions, FA. Serology: HI, SN, Elisa, DID. Differentiate from Egg Drop Syndrome, EDS-76.

Treatment

Sodium salicylate 1gm/litre (acute phase) where permitted - antibiotics to control secondary colibacillosis (q.v.).

Prevention

Live vaccines of appropriate sero-type and attenuation, although reactions can occur depending on prior immunity, virulence, particle size (if sprayed) and general health status. Maternal immunity provides protection for 2-3 weeks. Humoral immunity appears 10-14 days post vaccination. Local immunity is the first line of defence. Cell-mediated immunity may also be important.

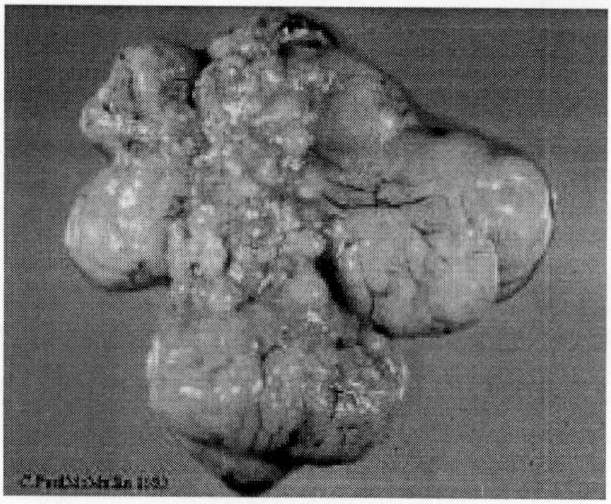

Fig: Flaccid Ovarian Follicles in a Broiler Parent Chicken Undergoing Challenge with Infectious Bronchitis Virus.

MYCOPLASMA GALLISEPTICUM INFECTION

A slow onset chronic respiratory disease of turkeys often with severe sinusitis and associated with Mycoplasma gallisepticum infection. It is seen worldwide, though in many countries this infection is now rare in commercial poultry. Morbidity is low to moderate and mortality low. The route of infection is via the conjunctiva or upper respiratory tract with an incubation period of 6-10 days.

Transmission may be transovarian, or by direct contact with birds, exudates, aerosols, and fomites. Recovered birds remain infected for life; subsequent stress may cause recurrence of disease. The infectious agent survives for only a matter of days outwith birds, although prolonged survival has been reported in egg yolk and allantoic fluid, and in lyophilised material. Survival seems to be improved on hair and feathers. Stress, malnutrition, intercurrent viral disease such as Newcastle disease (even lentogenic) and Turkey Rhinotracheitis are predisposing factors.

Signs

- Coughing.
- Nasal and ocular discharge.
- Swollen sinuses.
- Slow growth.
- Leg problems.
- Stunting.
- Inappetance.

Post-mortem Lesions

- Swollen infraorbital sinuses, often with inspissated pus.
- Airsacculitis.
- Pericarditis.
- Perihepatitis.

Diagnosis

Lesions, serology, isolation and identification of organism, demonstration of specific DNA (commercial kit available). Culture, of swabs taken from the trachea or lesions, requires inoculation in mycoplasma-free embryos or, more commonly in Mycoplasma Broth followed by plating out on Mycoplasma Agar. Suspect colonies may be identified by immunofluorescence.

Serology: serum agglutination is the standard screening test, suspect reactions are examined further by heat inactivation and/or dilution. HI may also be used. Suspect flocks should be re-sampled after 2-3 weeks. Some inactivated vaccines induce 'false positives' in serological testing. PCR is possible if it is urgent to determine the flock status. Differentiate from viral respiratory disease, especially Turkey Rhinotracheitis.

Treatment

Tilmicosin, tylosin, spiramycin, tetracyclines, fluoroquinolones. Effort should be made to reduce dust and secondary infections.

Prevention

Eradication of this infection has been the central objective of official poultry health programmes in most countries. These are based on purchase of uninfected poults, all-in/all-out production, and biosecurity. In some circumstances preventative medication of known infected flocks may be of benefit.

MYCOPLASMA MELEAGRIDIS INFECTION

A disease of turkeys characterised by respiratory and skeletal problems caused by Mycoplasma meleagridis. The organism has also been isolated from raptors, it occurs in most turkey-producing countries but is now much rarer in commercial stock. In adult birds though infection rates are high, morbidity may be minimal. Pathogenicity is quite variable. Mortality is low, though up to 25 per cent of infected birds show lesions at slaughter.

Infection is via the conjunctiva or upper respiratory tract with an incubation period of 6-10 days. Transmission is venereal in breeders, with transovarian and then lateral spread in meat animals. Infected eggs result in widespread distribution of infection and increased risk of further vertical transmission. The infective agent does not survive well outside the bird. Predisposing factors include stress and viral respiratory infections.

Signs

- Reduced hatchability.
- Slow growth.
- Leg problems.
- Stunting.
- Mild respiratory problems.
- Crooked necks.
- Infected parents may be asymptomatic.

Post-mortem Lesions

- Airsacculitis in infected pipped embryos and poults.
- Airsacculitis (rarely) seen in adult birds.

Diagnosis

Lesions, serology, isolation and identification of organism, demonstration of specific DNA (commercial kit available). Culture requires inoculation in mycoplasma-free embryos or, more commonly in Mycoplasma Broth followed by plating out on Mycoplasma Agar. Suspect colonies may be identified by immuno-fluorescence.

Serology: SAG used routinely - culture used to confirm. Differentiate from Mycoplasma gallisepticum, Mycoplasma synoviae, other respiratory viruses.

Treatment

Tylosin, spiramycin, tetracyclines, fluoroquinolones. Effort should be made to reduce dust and secondary infections.

Prevention

Eradication of this infection is also possible using similar techniques as for Mycoplasma gallisepticum. These are based on purchase of uninfected poults, all-in/all-out production, and biosecurity. Infected males are particularly prone to transmit infection and may warrant special attention. In some circumstances preventative medication of known infected flocks may be of benefit.

Vaccines are not normally used. Infected birds do develop some immunity. Birds infected from their parents seem to be immuno-tolerant and particularly prone themselves to transmit.

ORNITHOBACTERIUM INFECTION

Ornithobacterium Infection is an infection of chickens and turkeys with the bacterium Ornithobacterium rhinotracheale (ORT). This was first identified as a new disease syndrome of turkeys in Germany in the early 1990s. The slow-growing bacterium was named in 1994. It had been previously isolated in a number of other countries. The infection is common in chickens and turkeys. The severity of its effects depends on the pathogenicity of the particular strain and other risk factors such as viral infections, ventilation problems, age at infection etc.

Inoculation of fresh material from a case can reproduce lung lesions similar to those caused by Pasteurella multocida infection in previously uninfected turkeys over 10 weeks of age. It commonly exacerbates respiratory disease caused by pneumovirus infections in turkeys. In broiler chickens its main importance seems to be as a cause of airsacculitis in apparently healthy flocks that is only identified at slaughter. This can cause significant losses through condemnations. Important cofactors may include respiratory viral vaccines (Newcastle disease, Infectious Bronchitis), field challenge with respiratory viruses, Bordetella avium infection, and E. coli infections.

Some uncertainty exists about mechanisms of transmission. Within the poultry house it is likely to be by aerosols, direct contact and drinkers. There is some evidence that hatcheries may play a role in the epidemiology, perhaps through survival of the organism on shell surfaces or shell membranes. A range of sero-types have been identified. The range occurring in turkeys is wider than that seen in chickens.

Signs

- Coughing, sneezing.
- Reduced weight gain.
- Reduced egg production.

Post-mortem Lesions

- Airsacculitis, tracheitis, severe bronchopneumonia.

Diagnosis

Clinical signs and lesions. Confirmation is by isolation of the organism. Cultures from the trachea of birds showing typical signs are preferred. The organism grows slowly producing tiny colonies on blood agar. Growth is more rapid and consistent in an anaerobic jar. E. coli overgrowth may occur. It is a Gram-negative pleomorphic organism. Most isolates are oxidase positive and galactosidase positive Serology using Elisa tests has been used, preferably as a flock test comparing results before and after the challenge.

Treatment

The sensitivity of ORT to antibiotic is highly variable. Initially in Germany most strains were sensitive to amoxycillin, chlortetracycline but not to enrofloxacin. Amoxycillin sensitivity remains good, also most are sensitive to tiamulin. In France and Belgium most strains were sensitive to enrofloxacin. In the USA in 1998 all strains were sensitive to penicillins and many other microbials, though 54 per cent were sensitive to tetracycline, neo-mycin and enrofloxacin. Routine treatment - amoxycillin at 250 ppm in water for 3-7 days or chlortetracycline at 500 ppm for 4-5 days. Tilmicosin is also effective at 10-20mg/kg and should be used in the early stages of the disease.

Prevention

This is based on good hygiene, therapy and vaccination. Hygiene - it is very sensitive in vitro to a range of chemicals. ORT is a major problem on multi-age sites. Vaccination - there are issues relating to availability, regulation, cost etc. Some work has been done on live vaccine in the USA. An inactivated vaccine is licensed for broiler parents in Europe; it requires two doses. Some vaccines seem to have difficulty in producing a long-lasting serological response to ORT. Vaccination of breeder flocks to protect progeny has shown benefits in chickens but, because of the age of slaughter, this is unlikely to work in turkeys. Satisfactory disease control depends on good management and biosecurity.

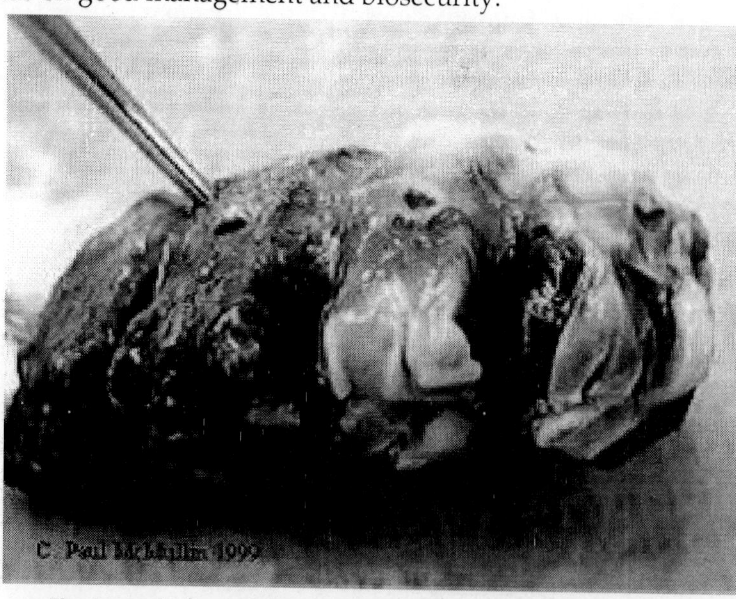

Fig: Severely Consolidated Lung from an Acute ORT Infection in 14-week-old Turkey Growers.

SALMONELLOSIS, PARATYPHOID INFECTIONS

Salmonellae bacteria other than the species specific sero-types S. Pullorum, S. Gallinarum, and also other than S. Enteritidis and S. Typhimurium (which are considered separately), are capable of causing enteritis and septicaemia in young birds. Sero-types vary, but S. Derby, S. Newport, S. Montevideo, S. Anatum, S. Bredeney are among the more common isolates. Even if these infections do not cause clinical disease, their presence may be significant with respect to carcase contamination as a potential source of human food poisoning. They infect chickens, turkeys and ducks worldwide.

Morbidity is 0-90 per cent and mortality is usually low. The route of infection is oral and transmission may be vertical as a result of shell contamination. Regardless of the initial source of the infection, it may become established on certain farms, in the environment or in rodent populations. Many species are intestinal carriers and infection is spread by faeces, fomites and feed (especially protein supplements but also poorly stored grain). Certain sero-types are prone to remain resident in particular installations (e.g. S. Senftenberg in hatcheries). The bacteria are often persistent in the environment, especially in dry dusty areas, but are susceptible to disinfectants that are suitable for the particular contaminated surfaces and conditions, applied at sufficient concentrations. Temperatures of around 80°C are effective in eliminating low to moderate infection if applied for 1-2 minutes. This approach is often used in the heat treatment of feed. Predisposing factors include nutritional deficiencies, chilling, inadequate water, other bacterial infections and ornithosis (in ducks).

Signs

- Signs are generally mild compared to host-specific salmonellae, or absent.
- Dejection.
- Ruffled feathers.
- Closed eyes.
- Loss of appetite and thirst.

Post-mortem Lesions

- In acute disease there may be few lesions.
- Dehydration.
- Enteritis.
- Focal necrotic intestinal lesions.
- Foci in liver.
- Unabsorbed yolk.
- Cheesy cores in caecae.
- Pericarditis.

Diagnosis

Isolation and identification. In clinical cases direct plating on Brilliant Green and McConkey agar may be adequate. Enrichment media such as buffered peptone followed by selective broth or semi-solid media (e.g. Rappaport-Vassiliadis) followed by plating on two selective media will greatly increase sensitivity. However this has the potential to reveal the presence of salmonellae that are irrelevant to the clinical problem under investigation. Differentiate from Pullorum/Typhoid, other enterobacteria.

Treatment

Sulphonamides, neo-mycin, tetracyclines, amoxycillin, fluoroquinolones. Good management. Chemotherapy can prolong carrier status in some circumstances.

Prevention

Uninfected breeders, clean nests, fumigate eggs, all-in/all-out production, good feed, competitive exclusion, care in avoiding damage to natural flora, elimination of resident infections in hatcheries, mills, breeding and grow-out farms. Routine monitoring of breeding flocks, hatcheries and feed mills is required for effective control. Infection results in a strong immune response manifest by progressive reduction in excretion of the organism and reduced disease and excretion on subsequent challenge. Vaccines are not generally used for this group of infections.

SPONDYLOLISTHESIS, KINKY-BACK

A complex condition of broiler chickens with a morbidity of 1-5 per cent and low mortality associated with rapid growth and possibly having a genetic component.

Signs

- Sitting on hock or rumps, legs extended forward.
- Use of wings to help in walking.
- May walk backwards.

Post-mortem Lesions

- Anterior-posterior rotation of the bodies of the last or penultimate thoracic vertebrae resulting in scoliosis just anterior to the kidney.

Diagnosis

Symptoms, lesions.

Treatment

None.

Prevention

Selection for satisfactory conformation in primary breeding.

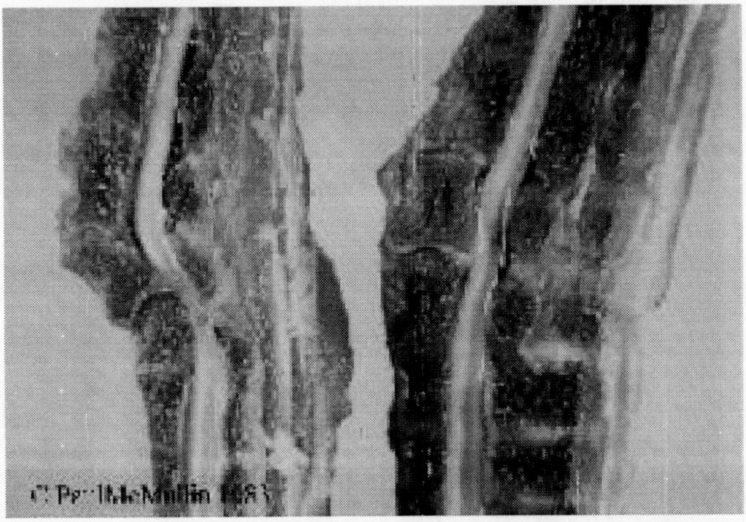

Fig: These are Cross-sections of the Spinal Column of 4-5-weekold Broilers. The Sample on the Right is Normal.

TRANSMISSIBLE ENTERITIS, BLUECOMB

Some coronaviruses involved in this condition are considered to be bovine coronaviruses (or closely related thereto); others are avian coronaviruses closely related to infectious bronchitis virus. The infection is seen in turkeys and sometimes pheasants. Morbidity is close to 100 per cent and mortality is 5-100 per cent. Transmission is lateral with birds and faeces, with rapid spread. The course of the disease is about 2 weeks and birds then remain carriers for months. The viruses survive in frozen faeces for months.

Signs

- Anorexia.
- Depression.
- Frothy diarrhoea.
- Subnormal body temperature.
- Darkening of the head.
- Loss of weight.
- Huddling.

Post-mortem Lesions

- Dehydration.
- Emaciation.
- Enteritis with petechial haemorrhages.
- Froth ingesta.
- Sometimes casts.
- Pancreas chalky.
- Urates in kidneys/ureters.

Diagnosis

Reproduction with filtered contents, isolation in turkey eggs, electron microscopy, immuno-fluorescence, Elisa. Commercial M4I IB Elisa will detect some infections.

Treatment

Warmth and good management, antibiotics, milk replacer, potassium chloride. Disinfect and rest houses for 3-4 weeks.

Prevention

All-in/all-out production, good hygiene and biosecurity, good management.

VISCERAL GOUT, NEPHROSIS, BABY CHICK NEPHROPATHY

Visceral gout is the deposition of white urates, which are normally excreted as a white cap on well formed faeces, in various tissues. Urates are also often deposited in joints and in the kidney. This condition can occur as an individual problem at any age. Outbreaks are seen in young chicks in the first week of life (baby chick nephropathy) or in flocks suffering kidney damage, or reduced water intake. All poultry species are susceptible. The kidney damage can arise from infection with certain strains of Infectious Bronchtiis virus, exposure to some mycotoxins or inadequate water intake (often because the birds have not adapated to a new type of drinker). Baby Chick Nephropathy can be due to inappropriate egg storage conditions, excessive water loss during incubation or during chick holding/transport, or inadequate water intake during the first few days of life. Very low humidity in brooding will also increase the likelihood of this problem. The timing of mortality is a reasonable guide as to the source of the problem. In Pekin/mallard ducks the condition is almost always due to inadequate water intake, whereas in muscovy ducks it is seen in breeders allowed to continue laying for over 24 weeks without a rest.

Signs

- Depression.
- Low feed intake and growth.

Post-mortem Lesions

- Chalky white deposits on pericardium, liver, air sacs, peritoneum.
- Similar deposits may be present in joints and are usually present in the kidney.

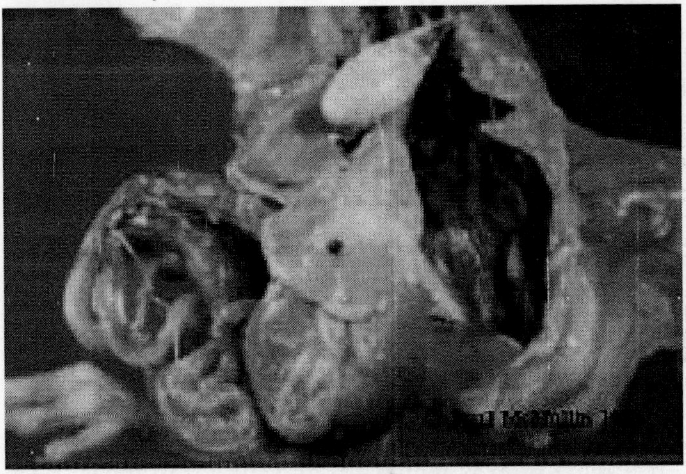

Fig: Severe Visceral Gout in a Young Chick.

Diagnosis

Lesions.

Treatment

This is based on correcting any management errors and encouraging water intake. Avoid any intentional or unintentional restriction in water intake. Sodium bicarbonate at 1g/litre water is mildly diuretic, however it could be counter-productive if water intake is in any way restricted.

Prevention

Careful monitoring of the conditions of hatching egg storage and incubation with a view to achieving a standard egg weight loss profile. Humidification of holding rooms and chick transporters may also be beneficial. Humidifiers in chick brooding areas are being used increasingly, especially where whole house hot air brooders are in use. Ample supplies of drinkers should be available and filled with water at house temperature prior to the arrival of the chicks.

□

5

Poultry Meat Industry

INTRODUCTION

The poultry meat industry accounts for approximately 10 per cent of the gross value of Australia's total livestock production and encompasses a variety of species, such as chickens, turkeys, ducks, quail, squab (pigeons), geese, pheasants, guinea fowl and other farmed avian species.

The chicken meat sector is the largest sector of the poultry meat industry, processing approximately 25-fold higher numbers of live birds and having 9 to 10-fold higher total retail value when compared to the non-chicken poultry meat sectors.

The turkey and duck sectors are the largest of the non-chicken poultry industry comprising 70 per cent and 21 per cent respectively.

It is estimated that 36 kg of chicken meat and chicken meat products are consumed in Australia per capita per annum. In comparison, per capita consumption of turkey and duck in Australia is estimated at 1.6 kg and 0.5 kg per annum, respectively.

Up to 70 per cent by weight of a live bird is recovered for human consumption. Of the products produced, 80 per cent are sold raw (as fresh or frozen whole bird or pieces), with the remainder as ready-to-cook or fully cooked value-added products.

THE CHICKEN INDUSTRY

Broiler Chickens

Virtually all chickens raised for their flesh (or "broiler chickens" as they are referred to by the meat industry), spend their lives crammed into massive, windowless sheds that typically hold as many as 40,000 birds each.

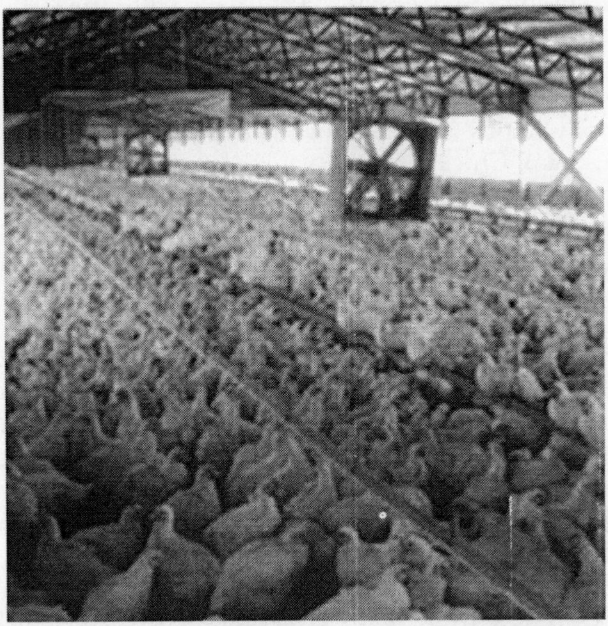

Chickens can function well in groups of up to about 90, a number low enough to allow each bird to find his or her spot in the pecking order. In crowded groups of thousands, however, no such social order is possible, and in their frustration, they relentlessly peck at each other, causing injury and death.

The intense confinement and extreme crowding on factory farms also results in unimaginable filth and disease. A Washington Post writer who visited a chicken shed said that the "dust, feathers and ammonia choke the air in the chicken house and fans turn it into airborne sandpaper, rubbing skin raw."

Michael Specter, a longtime staff writer for The New Yorker, also visited a chicken shed and wrote, "I was almost knocked to the ground by the overpowering smell of feces and ammonia. My eyes burned and so did my lungs, and I could neither see nor breathe .... There must have been 30,000 chickens sitting silently on the floor in front of me. They didn't move, didn't cluck. They were almost like statues of chickens, living in nearly total darkness, and they would spend every minute of their six-week lives that way."

These journalists could leave, but chickens are forced to breathe ammonia and particulate matter from feces and feathers all day long. Many suffer from chronic respiratory diseases, weakened immune systems, bronchitis, and "ammonia burn," a painful eye condition.

A 2006 study by Consumer Reports found that a staggering 83 per cent of grocery market chickens it tested were infected with either campylobacter or salmonella bacteria or both.The extremely high prevalence of dangerous contaminants in chicken flesh is due largely to the filthy conditions in the sheds where they are raised. On factory farms, they are fed large quantities of powerful antibiotics to keep them alive in conditions that would otherwise kill them: Chickens are given nearly four times the amount of antibiotics as human beings or cattle in the United States.

Chickens are also genetically manipulated and regularly dosed with drugs to make them grow faster and larger. The average breast of an 8-week-old chicken is seven times heavier today than it was 25 years ago. Because of this unnaturally accelerated weight gain, these very young birds frequently die of heart attacks and lung collapse, something that would almost never happen in nature. According to Feedstuffs, a meat-industry magazine, "Broilers now grow so rapidly that the heart and lungs are not developed well enough to support the remainder of the body, resulting in congestive heart failure and tremendous death losses."

In addition, chickens on today's factory farms almost always become crippled because their legs cannot support the weight of their bodies. In fact, by the age of 6 weeks, 90 per cent of broiler chickens are so obese that they can no longer walk. Many crippled chickens on factory farms die when they can no longer reach the water nozzles.

Breeder Chickens

The breeding animals who give birth to the 8 billion broiler chickens killed in the U.S. each year have been referred to as Gallus neglectedus, or "neglected chicken," by Dr. Joy Mench, a poultry scientist at the University of California, because their welfare is completely ignored.

Like the broiler chickens to whom they give birth, breeder chickens are confined to filthy sheds without access to sunlight, fresh air, or anything else that they would enjoy in nature.

When these birds are very young—usually just 1 to 10 days old—hot blades are used to cut large chunks off their sensitive beaks so that they won't peck each other out of frustration caused by the intense confinement. Sometimes their toes, spurs, and combs are also cut off. The birds are not given any painkillers to ease the agony of this mutilation, and many debeaked chickens starve to death because they are in too much pain to eat.

Breeder chickens are forced to live on factory farms for more than a year. Because they live so much longer, they face an even higher risk of organ failure and death as they grow larger and larger because of their manipulated genetics. In an attempt to fix this problem, the industry drastically limits the feed given to breeding birds, keeping the animals in a constant state of hunger and frustration.

When the birds drink more water to try to relieve their hunger, factory farm operators often reduce the available drinking water so that they won't have to clean up wet manure. Some farmers shove thin plastic rods through the delicate nasal cavities of male breeding birds. The rods stick out of both sides of their faces, preventing them from reaching through the wire barrier to eat the females' food.

After more than a year of deprivation and confinement, the bodies of these breeding birds are too worn out to produce enough chicks for the farmer to sell. Frail and exhausted, they are loaded onto trucks and sent to slaughter.

OVERVIEW OF THE POULTRY MEAT SUPPLY CHAIN

The structure and activities of the poultry meat supply chain can be divided into four stages: primary production, processing, retail and consumer.

Primary production includes all steps from the importation of fertilised eggs to the transport of live birds to the slaughter facility. The steps in the primary production of meat poultry. Differences in primary production between chicken meat and other poultry meat species are often observed in the type of housing/facilities used, composition of feed and age at which the birds are slaughtered. There are also different requirements for the importation of fertile eggs, with only chicken, duck and turkey eggs permitted to be imported into Australia.

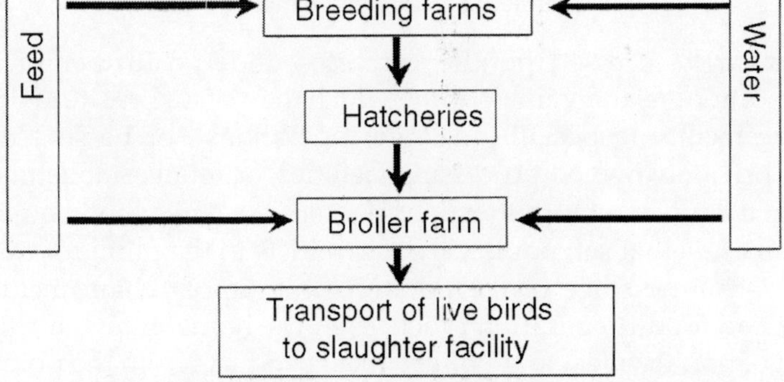

Fig: Stages in the primary production of meat poultry

Processing includes all steps from slaughter of live birds to the transport of poultry meat products to retail establishments. Poultry meat processing facilities vary in size between highly automated large, chicken processing facilities processing 4000 – 9000 birds per hour and smaller, largely manual or semi-automated facilities processing less than 1000 birds per day. The major steps in the processing of poultry.

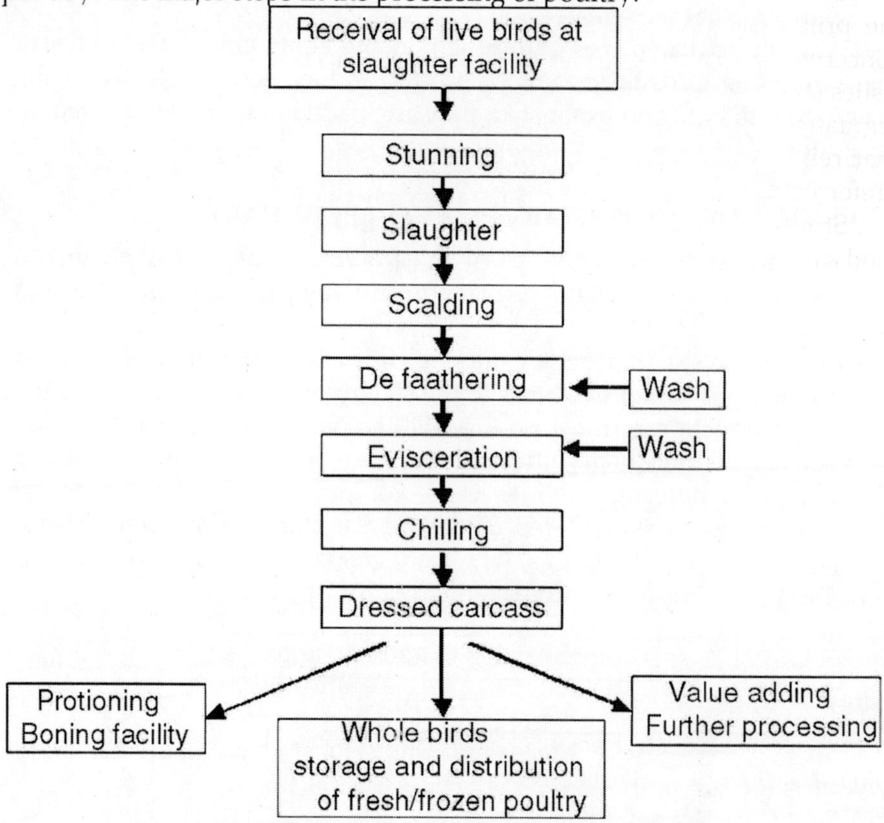

Fig: Stages in the processing of meat poultry

Increasingly, dressed poultry carcasses undergo further processing through portioning and value-adding which may occur on-site at the initial processing facility (especially in larger operations), or be sent to either separate, privately owned processing facilities, or retail establishments.

Retail includes restaurants, supermarkets, take-away food outlets, and other businesses that sell poultry meat products to the public.

The consumer stage of the poultry meat supply chain includes the handling and food preparation practices in the home. It also includes the transport of poultry meat and poultry meat products from the point of sale to the home.

SAFETY MANAGEMENT STRATEGIES IN THE POULTRY MEAT INDUSTRY

The safety of poultry meat and poultry meat products in Australia is controlled through a variety of regulatory and non-regulatory food safety management strategies which are described briefly in Attachment 2.

Current regulation of the poultry meat industry at the farm level of the primary production phase or poultry farm level is predominately concerned with animal disease control, animal welfare and environmental issues (air, water, soil, noise pollution). In addition to existing government regulations, the poultry meat industry has self-regulatory schemes in place that rely on voluntary compliance with codes of practice and industry preferred standards.

Strategies that exist at the poultry farm level which could impact on food safety include:

- Regulations for the importation of fertilised eggs and for the registration, sale and use of pesticides and veterinary medicines; and
- Regulations and non-regulatory codes of practice and guidelines for poultry feed (general stock feed requirements), poultry farming practices (including the layout and construction of farms), biosecurity, animal health and welfare and the transportation of live poultry.

The implementation of, and extent of compliance with these strategies varies depending of whether it is a legislative requirement or voluntary scheme and depending on the State or Territory.

Current State and Territory poultry meat regulation specific to food safety covers the slaughter, further processing, transport, and retail (including food service) of poultry meat products.

Objective

Poultry Meat is to cost effectively address the risk to public health and safety associated with the consumption of poultry meat and poultry meat products, in accordance with FSANZ's statutory obligations as set out in section 10 (1)

of the FSANZ Act:

- The protection of public health and safety;
- The provision of adequate information relating to food to enable consumers to make informed choices; and
- The prevention of misleading or deceptive conduct.

In developing and varying standards, FSANZ must also have regard to:

- The need for standards to be based on risk analysis using the best available scientific evidence;
- The promotion of consistency between domestic and international food standards;
- The desirability of an efficient and internationally competitive food industry;
- The promotion of fair trading in food; and
- Any written policy guidelines formulated by the Ministerial Council.

In addition, the Standard for Poultry Meat will aim to:

- Complement existing food safety management strategies to ensure complete coverage of the poultry meat supply chain;
- Be based on a comprehensive scientific risk analysis, using the best available scientific evidence;
- Be outcome-based and minimal effective regulation;
- Be nationally consistent thereby facilitating fair-trading in poultry meat and poultry meat products between States and Territories;
- Promote consumer confidence in an industry that is already highly regarded;
- Have the overall system costs commensurate with the assessed level of risk associated with the poultry meat industry and commensurate with the benefit to the poultry meat industry;
- Be consistent with internationally recognised poultry meat standards and internationally recognised principles of food safety;
- Encourage collaborative action among enforcement agencies to optimise the use of resources and to optimise the effectiveness of food safety standards in the poultry meat industry; and
- To have regard to the relevant policy guidelines formulated by the Ministerial Council and notified to FSANZ, regarding primary production and processing Standards.

Scientific assessment

As part of the FSANZ standard development framework, an assessment, Scientific Assessment of the Public Health and Safety of Poultry Meat in Australia, was undertaken in the context of the current regulatory and non-regulatory environment in the poultry meat industry and using international risk assessment protocols. The outputs of the scientific risk assessment were used to inform the development of risk management measures.

In particular, the assessment work identified:

- The food safety risks in the poultry supply chain; and
- Where these risks could best be managed in this chain.

The conclusions from the assessment were used to determine the gaps with the current management strategies in place, that is, where there are no or insufficient controls measures for an identified risk. Such gaps may be referred to as residual risk.

Scope of the Assessment

The risk assessment determined:

- The extent of food safety risk associated with the consumption of poultry meat and poultry meat products in Australia; and
- The factors along the poultry meat supply chain that have the greatest impact on public health and safety.

The risk assessment examined food safety hazards across the entire poultry meat supply chain– from importation of fertilized eggs through to consumption of poultry meat products. The microbiological hazards considered included Salmonella and Campylobacter species, pathogenic Escherichia coli, Staphylococcus aureus, Clostridium perfringens, and Listeria monocytogenes. Chemical hazards considered were agricultural and veterinary chemicals, contaminants, food additives and processing aids.

The assessment considered the major avian species consumed in Australia– including chickens, ducks, turkeys, geese, pigeons, quail, pheasants and guinea fowls. Wild caught birds (e.g. magpie geese and mutton birds) where processed in a registered establishment were also considered. However, ratites (emus and ostriches) were not included in this assessment as, they are processed using different methods to those used for the other avian species considered and the vast majority are processed in export-registered premises which are heavily regulated. Ratites will be considered in a subsequent primary production and processing standard.

As chicken meat represents the majority of poultry consumed, the risk assessment was largely informed by chicken meat data. The majority of the Australian data used was obtained from members of the poultry standard development committee. The hazards associated with chicken meat and chicken meat products were assumed to be similar to those associated with products from other poultry species, unless contrary data was available. This assumption was supported by the poultry standard development committee.

Main Findings of the Assessment

Salmonella and Campylobacter: Salmonella and Campylobacter are two of the most commonly reported causes of food-borne illness in Australia. Symptoms generally consist of self- limiting gastroenteritis, sometimes requiring hospitalisation. In a small proportion of cases, infection can lead to more severe, long-term illness such as septicaemia, reactive arthritis or Guillain Barré syndrome.

Based on epidemiological data, results from raw carcase microbiological surveys and outputs from the probabilistic model, there is reasonable evidence to indicate poultry is the vehicle for a proportion of salmonellosis and campylobacteriosis cases in Australia, however, due to a lack of quantitative data it is not possible to estimate the extent to which this is the case.

The following is a description of factors along the primary production, primary processing and food service/consumer handling and preparation stages that impact on the likelihood of contamination.

On-farm (from Uucleus Breeding Stock to Processing)

Contamination of poultry by Salmonella and Campylobacter on-farm is compared with another. Because of this, it was not possible to estimate the risk associated with various on-farm practices quantitatively. The report summarises current knowledge on practices that impact on contamination on-farm and highlights the differences between Salmonella and Campylobacter transmission at the primary production level.

There are a number of pathways by which poultry can become contaminated with Salmonella or Campylobacter. Some are more likely for one organism than for the other.

Contamination of birds by Salmonella on-farm can usually be traced to one or more of three factors: contaminated feed; environmental sources; and/ or vertical transmission from contaminated eggs. For Campylobacter, age of the birds and environmental contamination are the most important risk factors on-farm.

Based on domestic and international data, the major risk factors and their relative importance for Salmonella and Campylobacter contamination on-farm are shown in the following table. Significant variability and uncertainty is associated with the transmission of Salmonella and Campylobacter on-farm and the list should not be considered exhaustive nor the importance of each factor absolute.

Risk Factor	Increasing Importance			
Biosecurity				Salmonella Campylobacter
Vertical transmission from breeder flocks	Campylobacter			Salmonella

Positive chicks	Campylobacter			Salmonella
Previously positive flocks		Campylobacter		Salmonella
Litter/Insects		Campylobacter	Salmonella	
Contaminated Feed	Campylobacter			Salmonella
Age of birds		Salmonella		Campylo-bacter

Processing (from Arrival at Processing Plant to Poultry Meat Ready for Distribution)

The contamination of poultry meat is very much dependent on the status of the birds prior to slaughter and on operational hygiene during poultry meat processing. Processing converts live birds into meat and in doing so exposes the meat to contamination from the outside of the bird, the intestinal contents of the bird and the processing environment. Processing can be divided into a number of stages. Published studies on the effect of these stages on both the level and prevalence of Salmonella and Campylobacter on chicken carcasses are often conflicting, indicating a large amount of variability associated with each process. The following table highlights the typical effect of processing factors on the numbers of Salmonella and Campylobacter on chicken carcasses. It is recognised that individual plants or companies may perform these tasks differently and to different levels of hygiene.

Process stage	**Effect on contamination by Salmonella and Campylobacter**		
	Reduce	Minimal	Increase
Stun/Kill		Salmonella Campylobacter	
Scald - Low temperature	Campylobacter		Salmonella
Scald - High temperature	Salmonella Campylobacter		
De-feathering			Salmonella Campylobacter
Washing	Salmonella Campylobacter		
Evisceration			Salmonella Campylobacter
Washing	Salmonella Campylobacter		

Chilling – immersion		Campylobacter	Salmonella
Chilling – air		Salmonella	
		Campylobacter	
Portioning		Campylobacter	Salmonella

Generally, there is a tendency for the numbers of contaminated birds to increase during transport from farm to processing plants. The levels of Salmonella and Campylobacter on poultry carcasses generally fall during processing, although prevalence (i.e. proportion of contaminated birds) tends to increase, especially after evisceration. Chilling, under effective operation, usually results in a decrease in both numbers and prevalence. Although air chilling has been reported to reduce levels of Campylobacter contamination on carcasses, the extent of this is considered low.

Handling, Preparation and Consumption of Poultry Meat – a Quantitative Assessment

Available evidence indicates hygienic handling and proper preparation of poultry meat (either at home or food service) play a significant role in reducing the risk of food-borne illness associated with Salmonella and Campylobacter spp. This part of the risk assessment incorporates a quantitative model and was largely based on work undertaken by the FAO/WHO. Each module in the model deals with one or a set of specific factors that affect the levels and prevalence of Salmonella and Campylobacter. Parameters used in the model were based on published literature and/or data from government and industry surveys. An Excel based programme (@Risk, Palisade Corporation) was used to model the handling and preparation of poultry meat as well as the uncertainty and variability associated with the various model inputs. Uncertainty and variability were modelled using probability distributions.

The model considered factors such as:

- The prevalence and levels of contamination at the end of processing;
- The effect of freezing on the levels of Salmonella and Campylobacter;
- Growth of Salmonella during transport and storage (retail as well as home storage) of fresh chicken meat (no growth was assumed for Campylobacter);
- Possible cross contamination during preparation of foods;
- Reduction due to cooking; and
- The probability of illness from the consumption of contaminated poultry meat.

The output of the mathematical model simulating poultry meat transportation, storage and handling, is an estimate for the likely number of salmonellosis and campylobacteriosis cases resulting from consumption of poultry meat in Australia. The relevance of the risk estimate depends on (1) the extent to which the model represents precisely the practices in the various stages of poultry meat processing, handling and preparation, and (2) the availability of suitable and accurate data.

Due to a lack of both suitable and accurate Australian data across the entire model pathway, it is of little value in scientific terms to present final risk estimates in this document. More relevant to this risk assessment, however, is the impact on the estimated number of salmonellosis and campylobacteriosis cases by changing various model inputs.

A sensitivity analysis of the model inputs indicates that the probability of illness due to Salmonella contamination of poultry meat was most sensitive to the level and prevalence of the organism on the carcass at the end of processing, and its growth during distribution and storage. Improper thawing was also a significant factor. Cross-contamination and inadequate cooking were positively correlated with increased likelihood of illness.

For Campylobacter, the probability of illness was influenced by its level and prevalence at the end of processing and cross-contamination during preparation, e.g. not washing hands after handling raw poultry or using contaminated cutting boards to prepare other foods. Cooking adequacy was also influential on the final probability of illness.

The level and prevalence of both Salmonella and Campylobacter on carcasses at the end of processing had a large influence on the estimated number of illness. Based on the model, a ten-fold reduction in the level of contamination of Salmonella and Campylobacter at the end of processing resulted in a 74 per respectively. For both organisms there was a linear relationship between the prevalence at the end of processing and the final number of illness. In other words, halving the prevalence could halve the estimated number of illnesses. Halving the level of cross-contamination during preparation resulted in an 18 per cent and 27 per cent reduction in the estimated number of illnesses, respectively. Other scenarios were modelled, and the results are given in the body of the assessment.

OTHER MICROBIAL PATHOGENS

According to available data, there are no significant public health and safety risks resulting from pathogenic E. coli in poultry or poultry meat products in Australia. Although human pathogenic strains such as enterohaemorrhagic E. coli (EHEC) have infrequently been isolated from poultry internationally, there has been no documented case of food-borne illness due to E. coli associated with consumption of poultry meat in Australia.

The public health and safety risk due to S. aureus in poultry or poultry meat products is of minor significance. Although food-borne illness from ingestion of staphylococcal enterotoxin associated with the consumption of poultry meat has been documented, it is almost always due to contamination through post-processing handling.

Illness resulting from consumption of cooked poultry meat contaminated by S. aureus presents a risk due to the inactivation of competing microorganisms during cooking. Time and temperature abuse could allow growth of S. aureus that subsequently produce enterotoxin.

Although food-borne illness from consumption of C. perfringens contaminated poultry dishes has been documented, the public health and safety risk due to C. perfringens in poultry is of minor significance. Poultry meat can be contaminated with C. perfringens at the end of processing, however the levels are typically low, and significant temperature abuse and mishandling are required to allow growth of the pathogen to levels sufficient to cause illness. These risk factors occur primarily in the retail, foodservice/catering and home sectors, rather than the production and processing environments.

L. monocytogenes is often present on raw poultry meat but is rarely cited as cause of food-borne illness following poultry meat consumption. There is little evidence that multiplication of L. monocytogenes on raw poultry meat during storage is a major risk factor in human Listeriosis. L. monocytogenes is primarily a concern for ready-to-eat poultry meat products, particularly for susceptible populations. Contamination of ready-to-eat poultry meat may be as a result of inadequate heat treatment (i.e. cooking) or occur post processing, either directly from the processing environment or via cross-contamination at retail (e.g. sliced ready-to-eat meats). In the absence of competition with normal flora usually associated with raw poultry the organism can multiply, even when stored at <4°C.

Chemical Hazards

Given the data available for this review of chemical hazards in poultry and poultry meat products, the current regulatory measures outlined in the Code adequately protect public health and safety with respect to chemical hazards in poultry meat products in Australia. Data gaps relevant to the review of chemical hazards in poultry and poultry meat products have been identified.

Agricultural and Veterinary Chemicals

Maximum Residue Limits of the Code lists the maximum permissible limits for agricultural and pesticide chemical residues present in food. Contemporary survey results from the National Residue Survey (NRS) and Australian Total Diet Survey (ATDS) indicate that there is a high level of industry compliance with agricultural and veterinary chemical maximum residue limits (MRLs) in poultry meat products. These results indicate that dietary exposure to agricultural and veterinary chemicals through poultry meat products presents a negligible risk to the consumer.

Notwithstanding the results, there are concerns surrounding the adequacy of the agricultural and veterinary chemical testing regime particularly relating to the NRS. In 2002-2003 the NRS tested 165 chickens out of a yearly kill in excess of 400 million. Non-chicken poultry species were not tested. All tests were conducted on liver samples. Only five birds were tested for anticoccidials. Of specific concern was the breach of the MRL associated with the anticoccidial lasalocid. This data indicates either there was a sporadic breach associated with the use of the anticoccidial lasalocid or alternatively high-level breaches of MRLs associated with anticoccidials.

Contaminants

As part of the review of chemical hazards in poultry meat products, eleven contaminants with the potential to contaminate poultry meat were reviewed. FSANZ regulates the presence of contaminants. Two of the eleven contaminants reviewed (lead and polychlorinated biphenyls) have maximum limits (MLs) included in the Standard. Overall, none of the contaminants investigated demonstrated an immediate public health and safety concern in relation to poultry meat products,

However further investigation may be needed on the following contaminants:

- Arsenic – consistent presence of arsenic residues in poultry tissue and the absence of a permission for the anticoccidial roxarsone (4-hydroxy-3-nitrophenyl arsonic acid) in the Code; cent and 93 per cent reduce in the number of predicted cases of illness poultry at levels sufficient to contribute to an increased risk of dental fluorosis when combined with other sources of fluoride;
- Lead – reported high levels of lead in wild-caught birds, specifically the Magpie Goose (Anseranas semipalmata) harvested in the Northern Territory by local Aboriginal peoples. The use of lead shot will be phased out by 2005 in Northern Territory wetlands;
- Mercury – reported high levels of mercury in piscivorous waterfowl. There is currently an absence of data on mercury levels in mutton birds (Puffinus tenuriostris) to characterise the risk associated with consumption of this species.

The presence of dioxins and dioxin-like polychlorinated biphenyls were reviewed as part of the review of chemical hazards in poultry due to data made available through the National Dioxins Programme. The NRS provided data on 15 poultry meat samples and FSANZ on 11 poultry breasts. Though the data showed the dioxin dietary contribution from poultry meat to be low, the degree of testing is not sufficient to detect incidents of sporadic dioxin contamination in poultry in Australia.

Mycotoxins (aflatoxins, trichothecene toxins, zearalenone, ochratoxin A and fumonisin B1) were reviewed for their potential to contaminate poultry meat products via contaminated feeds. Though data on the carry-over of mycotoxins into poultry tissue is relatively scarce, the data consistently demonstrated low-levels of mycotoxin carry-over, insufficient to contribute substantially to total human dietary intake of these constituents.

Food Additives

The Standard, through Schedule 1, specifies permitted uses of food additives by food type for meat and meat type products (including poultry). The permissions for meat and meat type products relate mainly to preservative and colouring functions. There is a lack of data pertaining to the monitoring of food additives in poultry meat products.

Packaging

FSANZ regulates food contact uses of primary packaging materials. The Standard regulates food contact materials in general terms. The Standard does not specify individual packaging materials for food contact or how they are produced or used. FSANZ does not directly monitor for the migration of chemicals from packaging materials into food and as such the review is unable to characterise the risk associated with packaging materials in poultry meat products.

RISK MANAGEMENT (DETERMINATION OF RESIDUAL RISK)

Based on the available evidence, the scientific assessment concluded that chemical hazards from poultry meat and poultry meat products produced and processed under current food safety management strategies represent little risk to consumers. In addition, the probability of food-borne illness associated with pathogenic E. coli, S. aureus, C. perfringens and L. monocytogenes contamination of raw poultry meat and poultry meat products is also low. However, a potential food safety risk was identified for Salmonella and Campylobacter from consumption of poultry meat.

For each hazard considered within the scientific assessment, having regard to the current management strategies in place to address these hazards. A 'residual risk' is considered to be present when the current management strategies in place either do not address the identified hazard or do not adequately address this hazard.

The risk assessment identified a range of factors at the primary production, processing, retail and consumer stages that affect the prevalence and levels of contamination by Salmonella and Campylobacter on poultry and poultry meat products.

Primary Production

The risk assessment identified the main sources for Salmonella contamination at the primary production or poultry farm stage being the environment (i.e. lack of appropriate control measures), contaminated feed and contaminated eggs (i.e. vertical transmission), whereas for Campylobacter, the main source for contamination at the primary production stage is from environmental sources. Transport of birds to the slaughter facility was also found to increase prevalence of Campylobacter..

Contamination of Eggs with Salmonella

There are strict quarantine requirements for the importation of eggs and the hatching of those eggs to form the nucleus breeding stock. Due to the extent and comprehensiveness of these requirements, the importation of eggs and the hatching of those eggs to form the nucleus breeding stock are not considered to contribute to the residual risk.

The sanitation of eggs and monitoring of disease at breeding farms and hatcheries reduces the potential for microbial contamination of chicks. However, it must be noted that there have been reports of Salmonella being detected at these facilities. It is expected that environmental sources of contamination is the main avenue of Salmonella introduction into these facilities and subsequently into eggs.

Contamination of Poultry

Environmental sources were found to be a significant route for both Salmonella and Campylobacter introduction into breeding farms, hatcheries and broiler farms. The measures in place at these facilities to control the residual risk due to environmental sources are contained in voluntary industry codes of practice and guidelines: there are no regulations requiring farms to implement or comply with these measures.

These measures alone do not seem to be effective in reducing the likelihood of poultry being contaminated with Salmonella and Campylobacter spp. This may be because there is not sufficient market incentive for poultry farmers to implement the controls necessary to lower the likelihood of poultry being infected with these pathogens – the yield of poultry infected with these pathogens not being greatly affected, particularly with respect to Campylobacter.

This is a gap in the current food safety management strategies in place in the poultry meat industry, which is considered to contribute significantly to the residual risk.

One example of a voluntary industry code of practice is the National Biosecurity Manual for Contract Meat Chicken Farming, which covers facility, personnel and operational standards. This manual also has record-keeping templates for some farm practices. However, there is no information on the extent and effectiveness of the implementation of this and other codes of practice or guidelines, by industry. In addition, these codes of practices and guidelines were developed for animal health reasons and, although they may contribute to addressing food safety, were not designed with food safety as a focus.

In conclusion, the lack of enforceable national industry codes of practice is considered to contribute to the residual risk of poultry flocks becoming contaminated with Salmonella spp. or Campylobacter spp. at the primary production phase.

Contamination of Feed with Salmonella

Feedwasalsoidentifiedasapotentialsource for Salmonella contamination of poultry flocks. Both meat meal and grains can be contaminated with Salmonella and the heat treatment applied when the feed is pelletised is not effective at lowering Salmonella to safe levels if contamination levels are high. There are currently no existing nationally consistent regulations to prevent Salmonella contaminated feed being used to feed poultry. However, there are two strategies in place that address feed.

The Australian Standard has been adopted as a regulatory measure in a few States and Territories and requires that all rendering plants test for Salmonella weekly. A rendering plant must take corrective action after four positive samples in a window are detected, however rendered products can still be used to produce the feed that is fed to poultry. Feedmills operating under the industry-run FeedSafe accreditation programme, which also requires sampling and testing of poultry feeds for Salmonella. Although industry is monitoring this potential problem, the lack of measures to prevent Salmonella- contaminated feed being fed to poultry is considered to contribute to the residual risk and considered a gap in the food safety management strategies currently in place in the poultry meat industry.

CONTAMINATION OF POULTRY WITH CAMPYLOBACTER DURING TRANSPORT

Transportation of live birds to slaughter facilities was found to potentially increase the contamination of live birds with Campylobacter. Transportation of live birds is currently regulated under State and Territory animal welfare legislation and associated industry codes of practice. The legislation is concerned with factors such as water and feed requirements, shelter, loading and unloading birds and inspections.

There is a requirement in the Code of Practice for the Welfare of Animals- Land Transport of Poultry that transport cages must be 'thoroughly cleaned prior to use'. However, no further guidelines on how to achieve this requirement are provided and no outcome is stated.

Based on this information, the current food safety management strategies to address the transportation of live birds to slaughter facilities are not considered adequate to reduce the risk of birds becoming contaminated with Salmonella or Campylobacter spp.. This is a gap in the current food safety management strategies in place in the poultry meat industry.

Processing

The various State and Territory legislation requires that all poultry be processed (from slaughter to a finished product) under a comprehensive HACCP-based food safety programme. Under such a programme hazards are identified, evaluated and, if significant for food safety, controlled.

Various steps, in particular the scalding, defeathering, evisceration and chilling steps, in the processing of poultry and poultry meat products were identified in the risk assessment to impact on the prevalence and levels of Salmonella and/or Campylobacter spp.. It is expected that these steps are already monitored and controlled through the HACCP systems already in place in the processing sector. These existing requirements address the risk at the processing stage. The processing stage does not contribute to the residual risk provided the HACCP programme is effectively implemented and complied with.

Retail

The factors identified in the risk assessment that impact on Salmonella and Campylobacter contamination at retail and the existing requirements in the Code that address this risk. The existing requirements in the Code are consider adequate to address the risk at the retail level and ensure this stage does not contribute to the residual risk.

Table. The requirements in the Code that address the residual risk at the retail level

Risk factor	Requirement in the Code
The level and prevalence of these microbiological organisms entering retail establishments	The Code requires a food business to take all practicable measures to ensure that only food that is safe and suitable is received. However, a food business is limited as to what it can do on a practical basis when receiving potentially hazardous food (which includes all products containing raw and cooked meat). A business can really only check the food is protected from the likelihood of contamination and check that it is under appropriate temperature control. However, after receipt the food business will be able to assess the safety and suitability of the food. The food business must take all practicable measures to use only food that is safe and suitable. Safe and suitable food is food that will not cause illness or physical harm to a person eating it, provided that the food is used as it is intended to be used, and has not deteriorated, perished or contains a substance foreign to the nature of the food.

Conditions in which poultry meat and poultry meat products are distributed and stored at retail	The food storage clause lists the temperature requirements for potentially hazardous foods. There are similar temperature requirements for the distribution (transport) of food products. Product must also be protected from the likelihood of contamination during storage and distribution.
Improper thawing of frozen product	The Code requires the time that potentially hazardous food is kept at temperatures that support the growth of microbiological organisms when being thawed to be minimised. Frozen food must remain frozen.
Cross-contamination due to lack of hygienic handling during preparation	The Code sets out a number of requirements for the hygienic handling of food products. These include requirements for: • food handlers to take all reasonable measures not to compromise the safety and suitability of food; • food handlers to notify the business if he/she suspects he/she may have or could potentially (due to health) contaminate the food; • hygiene practices that minimises the contamination of the food; and • food businesses to have appropriate facilities to enable hygienic food handling practices.
Inadequate cooking of product	There are no specific requirements for cooking food products. However, a food business must ensure that if a food is to be cooked then the cooking step must be adequate to achieve a safe product (i.e. thoroughly cooked).

Consumer

The handling and preparation of poultry meat at the consumer stages of the poultry meat supply chain also have a significant impact on the risk of food-borne illness due to the consumption of poultry meat and poultry meat products. The main factors identified in the risk assessment that impact on contamination at the consumer level are:

- The level and prevalence of Salmonella or Campylobacter spp. on poultry meat products entering the consumers' home;
- Conditions in which poultry meat and poultry meat products are distributed and stored at retail and in the home;
- Improper thawing of frozen product;
- Cross-contamination due to lack of hygienic handling during food preparation; and
- Inadequate cooking of product.

If consumers handled and cooked poultry correctly, the residual risk from the primary production, processing and retail stages from raw poultry would be managed. However, as there are still cases of food-borne illness associated with consumption of poultry meat and poultry meat products in the home, it suggests that consumers are not able to fully manage the risks associated with poultry contaminated with Salmonella and Campylobacter.

Modelling within the scientific assessment clearly showed that reducing the level and/or prevalence of Salmonella and Campylobacter on poultry meat would result in a significant reduction in food-borne illness.

However, as the other stages of the poultry meat supply chain cannot completely eliminate all contamination of poultry from Salmonella and Campylobacter, it is important to reinforce to consumers the importance of handling and cooking poultry correctly.

The food safety management strategies for the consumer of poultry meat and poultry meat products are primarily education and information dissemination. These strategies are delivered through industry, governments, or non-specific consumer forums (i.e. associations, television programmes, magazine articles etc) however are generally not specific for poultry meat and poultry meat products.

The main messages conveyed to consumers are variations on the following six themes:

1. Keep hot food steaming hot;
2. Keep cold food refrigerated;
3. Cook food properly;
4. Separate raw and cooked foods;
5. Keep kitchen and utensils clean; and
6. Wash hands with soap and dry thoroughly.

Consider adequate to address the risk at the retail level and ensure this stage practices in the home undertaken for FSANZ suggests that most consumers report to be adhering to these practices (CRC, 2005). However, as food-borne illness in the home continues to occur, it is unclear to what extent these practices are actually applied.

The consumer stage is therefore considered to contribute to the residual risk.

Regulatory Problem

The scientific assessment identified a potential food safety risk from Salmonella and Campylobacter from consumption of poultry meat. The conclusion on the adequacy of current food safety management strategies to address the risk from these pathogens. In summary, the residual risk of Salmonella and Campylobacter contamination of poultry and poultry meat products is due to gaps in the current food safety management strategies at the primary production (breeding farms to the transport of birds to slaughter facilities) and consumer stages of the poultry meat supply chain. In contrast, the primary production stage prior to breeding farms, and the processing and retail stages do not significantly contribute to the residual risk, provided the current managements systems in place are implemented correctly and enforced.

Where gaps risks are identified there may be a number of options may be proposed to control those risks. The management options discuss strategies to address the identified residual risk within the scope of the FSANZ Act. There may also be other strategies that can be used to address the residual risk. For example, with respect to feed, the Meat Standards Committee and the Department of Agriculture, Fisheries and Forestry are already working on initiatives to improve the quality of the feed being produced. These initiatives are:

- The current review of the Australian Standard for the hygienic rendering of animal products through the Meat Standards Committee; and
- The Department of Agriculture, Fisheries and Forestry framework for updating control of animal feeds in Australia. The scope of this review would allow Salmonella in protein meals to be examined. FSANZ will contribute to this process, which will lead to a new national standard for animal feeds being developed.

RISK MANAGEMENT OPTIONS

The residual risk for each stage of the poultry meat supply chain, that is, primary production, processing, retail and consumer and concludes that there are gaps in the current management strategies to address this residual risk.

Various measures, both regulartory (standards) and non-regulatory (codes of practice, guidelines), can be used to address food safety risks. The decision as to what risk management measures are proposed takes into account the outcomes of the risk assessment process (what are the hazards and risks and where are they most effectively managed) and factors such as economic, social and technical feasibility.

Regulatory impact analysis is a critical part of the standards development process. Such an analysis must take into account the impacts on, and views of, all stakeholder groups affected by the proposed regulatory options – including industry, consumers, and governments. FSANZ must also ensure that the cost of the overall system is commensurate with the assessed level of risks and benefits.

These issues are considered in this report and will be further considered in the development of the Final Assessment Report and will address the requirements of the guidelines provided by the Council of Australian

Governments (COAG) (COAG, 2004). FSANZ must also ensure that the primary production and processing standard does not unnecessarily restrict trade and that it fulfils Australia's obligations to World Trade Organisation (WTO) agreements.

The development and discussion of the risk management options have been informed by:

- The evaluation of the food safety management strategies currently in place in the poultry meat industry;
- The outcomes of the Scientific Assessment of the Public Health and Safety of Poultry Meat in Australia (the risk assessment);
- Discussions with the Standard Development Committee and with other stakeholders, including the comments received in the submissions from the Initial Assessment Report; and
- An assessment of the regulatory impact.

FSANZ also commissioned Colmar Brunton Social Research to undertake research on the knowledge and awareness of safe food handling of poultry meat within the poultry meat industry, enforcement officers and consumers. The findings from this benchmark research have been used in the development and discussion of the risk management options.

Primary Production

The risk assessment identified breeding farms, hatcheries, broiler farms and the transport of birds to slaughter facilities as significantly contributing to the residual risk of Salmonella and Campylobacter contamination of poultry. Four risk management options to address this residual risk.

The four options are:

1. Maintain the status quo;
2. Encourage compliance with a code-of-practice (non-regulatory approach);
3. Require poultry growers to control food safety hazards and obligate poultry processors to ensure growers supplying them are meeting this requirement; and
4. Require poultry growers to implement a documented HACCP based food safety management system.

Status Quo

In maintaining the status quo, there would be no regulatory requirements for breeding farms, hatcheries, broiler farms or poultry transport operators to address food safety. However, these businesses could choose to follow industry based codes and would also be subject to any requirements placed on them by poultry processors. These measures alone do not seem to be effective in reducing the likelihood of poultry being contaminated with Salmonella and Campylobacter spp. This may be because there is not sufficient market incentive for poultry farmers to implement the controls necessary to lower the likelihood of poultry being infected with these pathogens – the yield of poultry infected with these pathogens not being greatly affected, particularly with respect to Campylobacter.

Without additional incentive, such as regulatory requirements on the primary production sector, the maintenance of the status quo is not likely to reduce the residual risk identified in the risk assessment. This means the levels of live birds contaminated with Salmonella and Campylobacter being supplied to poultry processors would remain the same. This affects the processor's ability to control the levels of Salmonella and Campylobacter during processing. While, the retailer or consumer could address these hazards through adequate cooking and correct handling of poultry, the current illness and outbreak data indicates this does not always occur.

Regulatory Impact – Industry

There would be no new costs for industry for maintaining the status quo.

Regulatory Impact – Government

There would be no new enforcement costs for government as there would be no government inspection of poultry farms. Enforcement officers would only enter poultry farms where it was suspected there were Salmonella positive flocks as a result of an outbreak investigation. Governments would continue to experience considerable costs in relation to the investigation of food-borne illness outbreaks.

Regulatory Impact – Consumers

The current levels of food-borne illness from Salmonella and Campylobacter to consumers and society would continue. An (as yet) unpublished report from OzFoodNet on food-borne disease associated with chicken meat and eggs, indicates that there were 52 reported chicken associated outbreaks between 2000-4 affecting at least 860 people, with 88 people hospitalised and one death (Kirk et al, 2005). In 1999, the then, ANZFA estimated an average cost of each food-borne illness case at $630 (ANZFA, 1999). This included both direct and indirect costs. Direct costs include those associated with medical care, loss of productivity, investigation of illness, loss of business and legal action. Indirect costs primarily include those associated with emotional loss. The Allen Consulting Group in its report on the costs and benefits of food safety management systems indicated that a range of literature suggests costs of between $4 and $6 million for the loss of life (The Allen Consulting Group, 2002).

The risk assessment concluded that the lack of food safety controls at the primary production stage contributes to the residual risk of food-borne illness due to the consumption of contaminated poultry meat and poultry meat products. Any lowering of this residual risk. Enforcement officer access to poultry farms would be restricted to when there is a reasonable belief that unsafe practices are occurring, by which time contaminated poultry would have already been processed and consumed. New costs for industry and government, the levels of food-borne illness from poultry contaminated with Salmonella and Campylobacter are likely to remain the same.

CODE OF PRACTICE – NON-REGULATORY APPROACH

The poultry farms would be encouraged to follow a code of practice that specifically addresses food safety issues at the primary production level. The food safety issues would need to cover those areas identified within the risk assessment as contributing

To the residual risk which were:

- The lack of measures on-farm to minimise environmental contamination of poultry from Salmonella and Campylobacter (including breeding farms, hatcheries and broiler farms);
- Measures to minimise Salmonella contaminated feed being fed to poultry; and
- Measures to minimise contamination of live poultry during transport.

The code of practice could be developed by industry, in conjunction with government.

The code of practice on the National Biosecurity Manual Contract Meat Chicken Farming, which is the main guide poultry growers currently refer to, with 65 per cent of growers indicating they adhere to it when prompted (Colmar Brunton Social Research, June 2005). However, the Manual primarily addresses animal diseases and welfare biosecurity measures and would need to be up-dated to cover all food safety hazards on poultry farms, particularly managing feeds, which is not specifically addressed.

There would need to be a high level of compliance with the code of practice to be effective at reducing the residual risk. This would be difficult to measure, as enforcement officers would have no power to inspect the farms to assess compliance.

Their powers would be limited. Processors could make compliance with the code of practice part of the contractual arrangements with the farm and check compliance. However, there would be no legal obligation on them to do so.

Regulatory Impact – Industry

The costs of compliance with a code of practice will depend on the degree to which procedures/practices on the farm would need to be modified to comply with the code of practice.

Regulatory Impact – Government

There would be no new enforcement costs for government as there would be no government inspection of farms.

Regulatory Impact – Consumers

The potential for the levels of food-borne illness from contaminated poultry and poultry meat to be lowered is dependent on the level of compliance with the code of practice. What this level would be is uncertain.

A voluntary code of practice that specifically addresses food safety risks has the potential to reduce the residual risk to public health and safety of poultry meat being contaminated with either Salmonella or Campylobacter spp. if it is applied.

However, the degree to which this residual risk can be lowered, as it is difficult to predict the percentage of farming operations that would comply with a code of practice. While poultry processors could require poultry farming operations to comply with a code of practice as part of a contractual agreement, this would not be a legal obligation.

It is reasonable to assume there would be a percentage of poultry farmers who would comply with the code of practice and correspondingly there would be a lowering of the residual risk. Therefore, greater benefits for consumers, where the residual risk is expected to remain the same. However, could be more costly to poultry farmers, as there may be costs associated with complying with the code of practice.

The Poultry Primary Production Sector to Control Food Safety Hazards

Primary Production and Processing Standard for Poultry Meat is adopted and requires:

- Businesses in the primary production sector to systematically examine all of their primary production operations to identify potential poultry food safety hazards and implement controls that are commensurate with the food safety risk; and
- A poultry processor to ensure only poultry is received from a grower who complies with the above requirement. A poultry processor would also be required to keep records to demonstrate compliance with this requirement.

The aims to recognise existing commercial arrangements between a poultry grower and a poultry processor. Poultry growers would normally be under a contract to supply a processor with the live birds, with the birds invariably being owned by the processor. For example, the chicken meat industry has advised that chicken which may not be grown under contract, i.e. where the processor is not also the owner of the chickens, is likely to be less than 1 per cent. Discussions with the game bird industry have also confirmed that growers are usually contracted to processors for the provision of birds.

Most poultry processors require poultry farms to meet food safety obligations as part of their contract of supply and audit the farms to ensure they are meeting these obligations, as 87 per cent of poultry growers indicated they adhere to contractual arrangements in relation to food safety (65 per cent unprompted) (Colmar Brunton Social Research, June 2005). Therefore, if this relationship between the grower and processor is recognised in terms of legal obligations, greater public accountability can be provided.

A greater potential to lower the residual risk from Salmonella and Campylobacter as it has legislative force. The enforcement agency can assess whether the processor is adequately monitoring the controls that address food safety hazards at the primary production level. It can also determine, by auditing records kept by the processor, whether the processor is inspecting the farm to assess the degree to which the farm is controlling its food safety hazards and whether it is following up areas of non-compliance. If the enforcement agency has any concerns with this arrangement, it can inspect the farm. Additionally, a primary production business could be prosecuted if it continued to follow unsafe practices.

Regulatory Impact – Industry

The poultry farming operations to address food safety hazards on farm by putting in place controls to minimise contamination of poultry from:

- Wild and domestic animals and birds;
- Insects and rodents;
- Drinking water;
- Feed and litter;
- Personnel; and
- Equipment.

These controls cover those areas identified within the risk assessment as contributing to the residual risk.

The specific practices a poultry farmer would be expected to implement for the above controls, that could incur a cost include:

- Protecting poultry from wild birds and rodents (this would require the shed to be wild bird and rodent proofed to the extent that is practicable and for pest control management to be in place);

- Providing clean continuous drinking water for the birds;
- Providing good quality feed (poultry to be fed feed that has been treated to reduce Salmonella levels to the extent practicable and stored so that it is protected from contamination from pests, wild birds, other livestock);
- Cleaning (and disinfecting) sheds in between each flock;
- Cleaning pickup equipment, crates and trailers (where the responsibility of the farmer);
- Providing clean or treated litter for each new flock (stored litter to be protected from contamination by birds, pests and other livestock);
- Providing protective boots and clothing for personnel and visitors;
- Providing hand washing facilities at sheds (this could be wipes or gels);
- Providing appropriate facilities to dispose of dead birds (sealed pest-proof containers or incinerators);
- Providing toilet and handwashing facilities for staff;
- Providing adequate facilities for waste disposal (including water disposal); and
- Keeping stocking densities to a level that minimises stress and susceptibility to microbial disease.

There are other practices a farm would need to follow that would have no or minimal costs associated with them such as:

- Keeping partial depopulation to a minimum (this is where part of a flock in a shed is separated for slaughter);
- Withdrawing feed for a time prior to slaughter to ensure the crop is empty;
- Cleaning up feed spills immediately;
- Minimising stress of birds during transport (this includes not overcrowding and handling birds with care during loading and unloading);
- Maintaining the farm in a clean and tidy condition;
- Separation of sick or dead birds from main flock;
- Ensuring farm staff do not have contact with other poultry, avian species or pigs;
- Limiting access to sheds; and
- Storing chemicals separately (away from feed, litter and poultry).

It would be expected that the vast majority of poultry growers are already complying, or are substantially complying, with these minimum requirements for food safety and therefore the proposed requirements. This expectation is supported by the benchmark research results quoted previously where 87 per cent of poultry farmers indicated they adhere to contractual arrangements in relation to food safety (65 per cent unprompted) and 65 per cent of growers indicating they comply with the National Biosecurity Manual for Contract Meat Chicken Farming, when prompted (Colmar Brunton Social Research, June 2005). This Manual covers the majority of areas listed above, with the exception of feed. This is also supported by industry who have advised that the biosecurity guidelines in the Manual have been in place for some years and stipulate practices in line with those necessary to meet the requirements.

The benchmark research also asked growers what sorts of things they did to reduce the risk of food-borne illness from poultry meat products. When asked spontaneously, growers most often mentioned that sheds are cleaned out between batches of birds (34 per cent), followed by maintaining a clean water supply (22 per cent). When prompted, most farmers (89 per cent and higher) indicated they do a wide range of activities to reduce the risk of food- borne illness from poultry meat products.

These activities and the percentage of prompted and unprompted responses, were:

- Rodent control is in place (99 per cent prompted, 10 per cent unprompted);
- A clean water supply is maintained for birds (98 per cent prompted, 22 per cent unprompted);
- Sheds are cleaned out between batches (97 per cent prompted, 34 per cent unprompted);
- Feed spillages are cleaned up immediately (97 per cent prompted, 8 per cent unprompted);
- Dead birds are disposed of in a biosecure manner (96 per cent prompted, 17 per cent unprompted);
- Foot baths are in place (93 per cent prompted, 31 per cent unprompted);
- Employees regularly wash their hands (90 per cent prompted, 10 per cent unprompted);
- Bird health is checked regularly (90 per cent prompted, 10 per cent unprompted);
- Sheds are left for 7-10 days between batches (89 per cent prompted, 8 per cent unprompted); and
- Wild Species are kept off the farm (89 per cent prompted, 9 per cent unprompted).

For poultry growers not currently controlling their food safety hazards, there are likely to be costs associated with improving their practices. There could also be costs associated with up-grading sheds and equipment if this is necessary to achieve hazard control. For example, if chickens are housed in sheds that cannot be proofed against rodents and wild birds and/or cleaned, they will need to be up-graded. One grower, who has recently built new sheds, indicated the cost was approximately $60 000 per shed (the sheds house 24 000 birds each).

A duck processor has indicated that of the 20 poultry farmers supplying birds, there is a possibility of three not meeting the requirements. However if an extended implementation period was provided, the costs per year to these producers would not be excessive.

To lessen the burden of cost for growers, an implementation period of two years should be provided.

The other costs that need to be considered are licensing and inspection fees. The government can inspect poultry primary production operations to assess whether growers are controlling their food safety hazards. However, it is expected that the enforcement of the requirement would be primarily through the processor, as the processor is required to ensure poultry is received only from a farming operation that is controlling its food safety hazards and must also keep records to demonstrate compliance with this requirement. The enforcement agencies have indicated they will limit their inspection of poultry farms to those occasions where there is concern that a farm may not be controlling food safety hazards. This could occur when:

- A farm is supplying a processor without a contract or the existing contract does not require adequate food safety controls to be in place on the farm;
- There is no or insufficient evidence that the processor is checking its farms to assess whether adequate food safety controls are in place;
- A processor has not satisfactorily followed up on unsatisfactory practices found to be occurring on its farms;
- Despite efforts on behalf of the processor, records indicate that a grower is not satisfactorily controlling its food safety hazards; and
- To follow up a suspected food-borne illness outbreak or a complaint.

Therefore, there will be some inspections at the primary production level. With respect to inspection costs,

Jurisdictions have indicated the following:

- Victoria will only inspect on farm if there is a concern with the arrangement between the processor and the farm and is proposing to absorb these costs;
- New South Wales may charge a license fee for each farm in the order of $200 annually to cover random checking of farms, as deemed necessary. If a farm needed follow up inspections because there were non-conformances it would be charged for this at approx $200 per hour;
- Queensland would inspect a farm if there was a concern but would not charge for this initial inspection. However, charges would apply if follow up inspections were needed at approx $200 per hour (this follow up inspection may be conducted by a third party auditor);
- In South Australia farms may need to be accredited (or licensed), with the charge being approximately $120/year. South Australia would restrict auditing of farms to where corrective action by the processor has been unsuccessful. In such cases, the farm would pay for the audits until compliance is achieved (current rate is $128/hr). The length of the audit would depend on the nature of the non-compliance and the size of the farm;
- Tasmania is not proposing to charge license fees on farms. It proposes to enforce this requirement through the auditing of the processor and if it is necessary to go back on farm, would recoup these costs from the processor; and
- Western Australia is not anticipating inspecting or auditing farms on a routine basis. Farms may be inspected when evidence held by a processor indicates there is an issue on farm that is not being adequately addressed. At the present time, Western Australia has no scope to charge licence fees or charge for inspections and audits. However, this may change in the future.

The Northern Territory and the Australian Capital Territory do not have any farming operations growing poultry for sale for human consumption.

Regulatory Impact – Government

The enforcement agencies have indicated that the main costs will be associated with the physical inspections that need to be conducted and will include:

- Staff time to inspect farms and follow up on areas of non-compliance;
- Maintaining either an electronic database or paper records of farms and inspection results;
- Transport to and from farms; and

It is not expected that there will be additional costs to set up a database as existing systems can be used for this new function. The costs associated with licensing and inspection/audit fees, as outlined above under the discussion on the regulatory impact to industry. Therefore, the impact of these changes on government is likely to be low.

Regulatory Impact – Consumers

The regulatory component will give greater public accountability to existing arrangements that are in place between poultry processors and the growers that supply these processors with live poultry. If there are any concerns that this arrangement is not working and hence food safety hazards are not being controlled on farm, government will be able to intervene. Therefore, it is expected has a greater potential to lower the residual risk of poultry contaminated with Salmonella and Campylobacter reaching the consumer where no government checking is recommended. If the likelihood of poultry being contaminated with Salmonella and Campylobacter is reduced, it follows that the incidence of food- borne illness occurring from these pathogens will also be reduced. This will directly benefit consumers. However, this benefit may come at a cost to consumers if the poultry industry charges consumers more for poultry meat and poultry meat products to recoup any additional costs it incurs.

It is anticipated that this government intervention will result in improved food safety practices, thereby lowering the residual risk to consumers of suffering food-borne illness from contaminated poultry meat and poultry meat products. However, this lowering of the residual risk comes at a cost. The likely costs to poultry primary production operations are:

- Costs to improve food safety practices and up-grade facilities and equipment where necessary to meet the new requirements;
- License or accreditation fees in some jurisdictions (in the order of $120-$200 per annum); and
- Costs associated with auditing/inspection if there are concerns the farming operation is not meeting its legal obligations. Costs will include direct costs for the audit/inspection and indirect costs such as staff time spent with the auditor/inspector.

It is expected that the vast majority of primary production operations would already be meeting the food safety practices and therefore the cost impact is expected to be minimal. While the licence/accreditation fees represent new costs (for those poultry growers located in jurisdictions where these will apply), the audit/inspection fees can be avoided if the processor and the grower adequately meet the legal obligations.

Documented Haccp Based Food Safety Management System

A poultry grower would be required to implement a documented food safety management system that effectively controls the hazards.

A poultry grower could be taken to comply with this requirement if it implements:

- A Codex Hazard Analysis Critical Control Point (HACCP) food safety management system; or
- A HACCP based food safety management system recognised by the Authority (this would include recognised industry developed programmes).

The HACCP programme would need to:

- Identify potential food safety hazards that may be reasonably expected to occur on the farm;
- Identify where each of these hazards can be controlled and how they will be controlled; and
- Indicate what corrective actions will be taken if a hazard is found not to be under control.

The programme would need to be fully documented and records would need to be kept to demonstrate compliance with this programme, for example, pest control records, monitoring control measures and corrective actions taken.

Regulatory Impact – Industry

In addition to the compliance costs, the poultry grower would also incur the following costs:

- HACCP training for management and staff in supervisory positions;
- Management time to write the programme and to pay consultants to assist with this task;
- Once the programme is written, training of all staff on how to comply with the HACCP programme;
- Possible employment of additional staff, such as a quality control manager, to assist with these tasks;
- Ongoing costs of having the programme audited;
- Ongoing costs of reviewing the programme to ensure its adequacy;
- Ongoing costs of amending the programme when practices on the farm change;
- Training for new staff and up-dating all staff on any changes to the HACCP programme; and
- Keeping records to demonstrate compliance with the programme.

The cost of developing and implementing a HACCP programme for a duck processor has been estimated at approximately $100,000 to $150,000.

The above costs could be significantly reduced where is a specific guideline is available for poultry farming operations to use to assist in developing the HACCP programme for the business. The Australian Chicken Meat Federation (ACMF), the peak industry body for the chicken meat industry, is finalising such a guideline, Food Safety HACCP Programme for the Chicken Meat Industry. This Programme includes generic HACCP programmes for the entire chicken meat industry – from farming through to processing, including feed mills, hatcheries, breeder farms, broiler farms and processing plants. The ACMF is proposing to circulate copies of this programme to the entire chicken meat industry and run training workshops. It is not yet clear how applicable this guideline will be for non-chicken poultry.

While recognising that guidance material such as that being finalised by ACMF would significantly reduce the costs to poultry growers, the costs associated will still be higher. It is expected that the majority of farming operations would already be complying with the proposed requirements. However, most farming operations do not have HACCP programmes in place and therefore would incur costs to develop and implement such a programme to comply. There would also be the ongoing costs to comply with the programme, maintain it and have it audited. These costs are also likely to be prohibitive to a greater percentage of growers and therefore it is expected that a larger percentage of growers would close their businesses.

Regulatory Impact – Government

The most costly for government to implement. There would be initial costs in ensuring HACCP programmes developed by primary production businesses met acceptable standards and assistance and guidance to poultry farms.

All farms would need to be regularly audited to ensure compliance with the food safety programme requirement. Government could employ or train staff to perform this auditing function and/or approve third-party auditors to carry out this function. Even if the enforcement agency utilises third-party auditors, it will incur the cost of managing the administration required to ensure all poultry farms are regularly audited and non-conformances are followed up satisfactorily. The additional costs to government are likely to be recouped through licensing fees and auditing fees, if government officers carry out the audits. These costs will be higher than those indicated.

Regulatory Impact – Consumers

In respect to lowering poultry contamination with Salmonella and Campylobacter, as it would more actively and comprehensively require primary production operations to control food safety hazards. However, this benefit is likely to come at a greater cost. The additional costs to growers to comply with the HACCP programme proposed are likely to be passed on to the consumer and the resultant increases in the price of poultry meat and poultry meat products are expected to be higher than the minimal rises.

The highest costs for poultry growers, as they would need to develop and implement a documented HACCP programme. There would also be significant ongoing costs to comply with the programme (in terms of record keeping), to maintain it and to have it regularly audited. Though the developmental costs could be lowered where appropriate guidance material and assistance is available, the overall cost is expected to be much higher. These costs could be prohibitive to a significant number of poultry growing operations, causing these operations to be either sold or closed.

While compliance costs are expected to be higher, would be the most effective in reducing the residual risk of poultry being contaminated with Salmonella and Campylobacter. As additional costs to industry are normally passed on to the consumer, it is uncertain how much more the consumer is willing to pay for potentially safer food.

Preferred Option

The preferred option as it represents the most cost effective way of addressing the residual risk at the primary production stage of the poultry meat supply chain. To strengthen existing arrangements in place between a processor and farms that supply this processor by legally obligating poultry growers to control their food safety hazards and for the processor to demonstrate that its growers are meeting this obligation.

This enables the government to scrutinise these arrangements and to intervene where necessary. The resultant improved poultry growing food safety practices should flow on to a lowering of the residual risk to consumers. The costs associated are considered minimal, as the vast majority of poultry primary production operations are reportedly already controlling their food safety hazards.

The residual risk from poultry primary production operations identified within the risk assessment, thereby representing no benefit to consumers. There would be no change in the incidence of food-borne illness due to the consumption of poultry meat and poultry meat products and there would be no change to the current arrangements for poultry primary production.

In terms of the incidence of food-borne illness, an (as yet) unpublished report from OzFoodNet on food-borne disease associated with chicken meat and eggs indicates that between 2001-4, there were 52 chicken-associated outbreaks affecting at least 860 people, with 88 people hospitalised and one death (Kirk et al, 2005). This does not include non-outbreak associated illness, that is, sporadic occurrences related to the consumption of chicken meat and eggs.

The residual risk but the degree to which this residual risk can be lowered, as it is difficult to predict the percentage of poultry primary production operations that would comply with a code of practice. While poultry processors could require poultry growers to comply with a code of practice as part of a contractual agreement, there would be no public accountability, through government inspection/audit to assess the effectiveness of this arrangement. Therefore predicted to be more effective at lowering the residual risk.

Processing

In March 1995, the (then) Agriculture and Resource Management Council of Australia and New Zealand determined that aspects of all existing national meat industry codes relevant to human health would be mandated by amendment of legislation in all States and Territories. This decision was given effect by appointment of a Steering Group, which reviewed existing codes of hygienic practices (in relation to meat) to express mandatory national standards in outcome terms. The mandatory requirements were specified within Australian Standards and require process control to be achieved through the application of HACCP methodology as defined by the Codex Alimentarius Commission.

The Australian Standard requires poultry processors to develop and implement HACCP programmes. This programme must address the food safety hazards associated with the processing of poultry. The Australian Standard for poultry also requires businesses to comply with specific requirements relating to the design and construction of the premises, the processing of poultry, health and hygiene requirements and cleaning and sanitising.

The development of a national standard for poultry primary production and processing will enable the food safety hazards associated with the entire poultry meat supply chain (from the farm to the consumer) to be addressed within the one regulatory document i.e. the Food Standards Code. The risks from the processing stage of this chain can be addressed by the Standard for Poultry Meat,

Requiring poultry processors to:

- Develop and implement a documented HACCP based food safety management system as currently required under State/Territory legislation which mandates compliance with the AS 4465; and
- Food Premises and Equipment of the Code (the requirements within these Standards reflect the requirements within the existing Australian Standard for poultry for the design and construction of the premises, health and hygiene and cleaning and sanitising).

To ensure that the documented food safety management system addresses and controls the main hazards associated with the consumption of poultry meat, they should be specified within the Standard for Poultry Meat.

These hazards are:

- The removal of unacceptable poultry prior to slaughter and unacceptable carcasses during processing;
- The minimising of contamination of poultry, carcasses and poultry meat; and
- Minimising the levels and growth of pathogenic microorganisms potentially present on the poultry carcass or poultry meat.

The scope of activities to be covered within the documented food safety management system should be consistent with AS 4465. This means it should cover the primary processing of poultry (from holding of poultry before slaughter to carcass stage and deboning and portioning). It should also cover any further processing of poultry undertaken by a poultry processor such as marinating, crumbing, cooking and packaging. However, it should not cover food businesses handling poultry not currently covered by AS 4465, which are those within the retail/food service sector.

A specific requirement for poultry processors to maintain sufficient records to identify the immediate supplier and immediate recipient of poultry or poultry meat products for the purposes of ensuring the safety of the poultry meat products, has also been included in the proposed Standard. This is an important component of a food safety management system to enable tracing when product becomes contaminated. It enables contaminated product to be recalled and also assists in determining the cause of the contamination, such as a particular farm supplying contaminated poultry.

The Standard will need to be supported by a comprehensive interpretive guide that explains the intent of these requirements and in doing so, carries across the detailed food safety information contained within the AS 4465. The interpretive guide will also provide further detail on the controls that are critical to the safe production of poultry, as identified within the risk assessment. The poultry industry may also develop specific guidance material, for example, the guideline already being developed for the chicken meat industry by the Chicken Meat Federation, Food Safety HACCP Programme for the Chicken Meat Industry.

The requirements in the AS 4465 that do not relate to food safety such as animal welfare and occupational health and safety matters will need to be addressed through other mechanisms. The Food Regulation Standing Committee (FRSC) Primary Production and Processing Working Group has begun discussions on possible transitional issues in relation to the incorporation of the food safety elements of AS 4465 into the proposed Standard for Poultry Meat.

Regulatory Impact

There are four main requirements proposed for poultry processors:

1. develop and implement a documented HACCP based food safety management system as currently required under State/Territory legislation which mandates compliance with the AS 4465;
2. to ensure poultry farmers supplying poultry are controlling food safety hazards (to support the requirement on poultry farming operations); and
3. maintain sufficient records to enable the traceability of poultry and poultry meat products, where necessary for food safety.

A HACCP Based Food Safety Management System

There is no regulatory impact as this is a current requirement within State/ Territory legislation, which mandates compliance with AS 4465. This Australian Standard already requires poultry processors to develop and implement a HACCP based food safety programme.

There is no regulatory impact as the requirements within these Standards reflect those within AS 4465, which is mandated under State/ Territory legislation.

Requirement to Ensure Poultry Farmers Supplying Processors

The preferred risk management option for the primary production phase of the poultry meat supply chain, recommends that poultry processors be required to ensure that poultry growers supplying poultry are controlling food safety hazards.

The enforcement agencies that will be responsible for enforcing this requirement have indicated they will audit the processor's records to assess whether systems are in place to ensure poultry growers are controlling food safety hazards. If a processor is not currently monitoring poultry growers to assess compliance with contractual agreements, this requirement will mean additional costs.

Costs will include:

- Having access to appropriately skilled staff to assess compliance on poultry farms;
- Keeping records of farm compliance; and
- Following up areas of non-compliance.

Some of the smaller processors purchase poultry from the larger poultry companies and not directly from growers. They would therefore not be responsible for inspecting these growers. In such cases, the processor in question would need to obtain documented evidence from the company who has direct responsibility for the farms, that food safety hazards are being controlled. The larger players in the poultry industry have indicated they already regularly check their growers to assess whether they are controlling food safety hazards and therefore this requirement will have little impact. The enforcement agencies have also indicated that the time needed to assess additional records required by this requirement will add minimal costs to the overall auditing cost (in the order of 1 per cent).

The poultry processors on whom this new requirement will have most impact are those not currently conducting regular monitoring of poultry growers. While this represents a small percentage of the industry, this will have a financial impact on the affected processors. One such processor has indicated this new requirement will cost the business an additional $50 000 per annum. This cost could not be absorbed by the business and hence it would be passed on to the consumer through increased prices.

To avoid this cost, the requirement on poultry processors to ensure its poultry growers are controlling food safety hazards could be deleted and instead government would need to regularly inspect poultry farms to assess compliance. This would be duplicative as the majority of the poultry industry has indicated it already carries out this function and would continue to do so even if government inspected poultry growing operations.

The requirement for poultry processors to ensure poultry growers are controlling food safety hazards reflects current industry practices for the majority of the industry. Therefore, the overall additional costs on the industry and therefore to the consumer are expected to be minimal.

Retail

The risk assessment concluded that the potential risks from poultry at the retail stage of the poultry meat supply chain are adequately addressed through the requirement. Although the risk management for the retail stage remains unchanged, FSANZ will reiterate the importance of effective implementation requirements to retailers as part of the communication strategy for the primary production and processing standard for poultry meat.

Consumer

The risk assessment concluded that improvements in the way in which consumers handle and cook poultry would significantly lower the levels of illness. To lower the risk of consumers becoming ill from Salmonella and Campylobacter they need to:

- Keep raw poultry refrigerated and well away from cooked and other ready-to-eat foods;
- After handling raw poultry, wash and dry hands thoroughly;
- Cook the poultry thoroughly so that juices run clear and no pink is visible; and
- Ensure that the cooked poultry does not become contaminated with juices from the raw poultry by ensuring only clean, dry utensils and equipment are used for the cooked poultry.

The Food Safety Information Council, the Australian organisation with primary national responsibility for conveying food safety messages to consumers, aims to improve consumer's knowledge of how to handle, store and cook food safely. However, the food safety messages it promotes are general and not specific to poultry, for example, 'Cook food properly' and 'Separate raw and cooked food'.

To reduce the risk that raw poultry poses to consumers, there may be a need for more specific poultry food safety messages for consumers. One of FSANZ's functions, in cooperation with the Australian states and territories and New Zealand, is to help develop food education initiatives, including the publication of information to increase public awareness of food standards and food labels. Initiatives could include information targeted to specific sub- populations of the community (e.g. allergen suffers, vulnerable populations etc). Education raises awareness and increases understanding of food regulations, making them more effective, thereby making the food supply safer. FSANZ 's capacity is reduced if the agency works by itself in this area. The Poultry CRC may be an avenue to progress this through their programme of improved education and skills of staff at all levels of the industry.

Consultation

In addition to statutory consultation, that is the consultation required of FSANZ under the FSANZ Act, further consultative mechanisms have been built into the development process for the Primary Production and Processing Standard for Poultry Meat. Additional consultation reflects the recognition that close consultation with industry, regulators and consumers is needed throughout the development of the Standard. This is considered particularly important as the setting of primary production and processing standards is a new function of FSANZ.

Accordingly, in the early stages of standard development, the level of awareness of FSANZ processes in the community and within the primary production sector may be minimal.

As part of FSANZ's statutory consultation, the Initial Assessment Report was released for a six week public comment period from 26 May 2004 until 21 July 2004.

Minimisation of pathogen load at all steps of the supply chain

Although many submitters acknowledged inappropriate food safety practices by consumers, they believe that all sections of the poultry meat supply chain should be responsible for reducing the pathogen load in poultry and poultry meat products so as to minimise the impact of inappropriate handling and cooking at the consumer level of the supply chain.

Education

Many submitters suggested a need for more consumer education programmes, as ultimately consumers are able to reduce the potential for food- borne illness by appropriate cooking of poultry meat products and implementation of measures to reduce cross-contamination. FSANZ is working with industry through the Poultry Cooperative Research Centre to develop an appropriate consumer information package.

Strategies to Support the Standard for Poultry Meat

A number of submissions from consultation on the Initial Assessment Report emphasised that an essential part of the standard will be the guides that will accompany it. These guides could include an interpretive guide which describes each provision in the standard and an 'industry guide' which details the processes and procedures that an operator could use to meet the standard. Submitters believe such guides are essential for consistency in enforcement, compliance and food safety practices within the poultry meat industry.

FSANZ will develop an interpretive guide to the Standard for Poultry Meat in consultation with the Standard Development Committee. The guide will explain the requirements of the Standard and briefly summarise other requirements in the Code that apply to poultry meat. As has been the case with previous food safety standards, FSANZ would develop an interpretive guide for dissemination to enforcement agencies prior to the standard coming into effect.

The Australian Chicken Meat Federation has recently completed the development of a guideline, Food Safety HACCP Programme for the Chicken Meat Industry to provide specific guidance to the chicken meat industry on developing HACCP programmes. This would assist the chicken industry meet the legal obligations being proposed within this report by assisting:

- Processors to develop HACCP based food safety management systems; and
- Poultry primary production businesses identify and control their hazards.

The Australian Chicken Meat Federation proposes to run workshops in every State and Territory on this guideline programme.

Consumer Education

Many submitters felt that there should be a consumer education programme to accompany the standard, as ultimately consumers are able to reduce the potential for food-borne illness by appropriate cooking of poultry meat products and implementation of measures to reduce cross-contamination.

World Trade Organization (WTO)

As members of the World Trade Organization (WTO), Australia and New Zealand are obligated to notify WTO member nations where proposed mandatory regulatory measures are inconsistent with any existing or imminent international standards and the proposed measure may have a significant effect on trade.

The proposed Standard for poultry meat will have implications for imported product. Notification will therefore be made in accordance with Australia's obligations under Sanitary and Phytosanitary Measure (SPS) Agreement. This will enable other WTO member countries to comment on proposed changes to standards where they may have a significant impact on them.

EVALUATION OF OTHER REQUIREMENTS FOR POULTRY MEAT IN THE CODE

As part of the development of the Standard for Poultry Meat, an evaluation of other poultry requirements in the Code was undertaken.

Eviscerated Poultry

Evisceration is the process for removing the crop, intestines and other internal organs from the poultry carcass. As some of these organs can be highly contaminated with microorganisms such as Salmonella and Campylobacter, evisceration was considered in the assessment of the risk to public health and safety to have the potential to significantly contribute to carcass contamination. The significance of evisceration is recognised under State and Territory legislation where the processing of poultry must include evisceration.

Poultry in the form of an eviscerated carcass may include the gizzard, heart, liver, neck or a combination thereof.

As the Australian Standard requires the evisceration of all poultry and the food safety elements of this Standard are being transferred to the Poultry Meat Standard, it is proposed that this clause be deleted from the Code. Partly eviscerated poultry has the potential to be highly contaminated with pathogenic bacteria and therefore poses an unacceptable risk to consumers. The Australian Standard or on the jurisdictions as deletion brings the Code into alignment with requirements jurisdictions currently enforce.

Limit on Fluid Loss in Thawed Poultry

During the processing of poultry, water is used for washing and chilling, which results in the absorption or take up of water by the skin or muscle tissue of carcasses. This take up of water contributes to a loss of fluid that occurs when frozen poultry is thawed.

This limit was set in 2000 as part of the process of developing the meat standard for the joint Australia New Zealand Food Standards Code. Initially it was proposed that the limit of fluid loss from thawed poultry be 80 g/kg (8 per cent), the limit in Australia at the time.

Eight submissions were received of which 5 supported the proposal to limit fluid loss to 8 per cent, one questioned whether the issue of fluid loss could be handled as a fair trading issue and one proposed a level of 6 per cent because it was the level in the New Zealand Food Regulations and reflected practice at that time. From these submissions, FSANZ (then ANZFA) proposed to lower the limit from 8 per cent to 6 per cent and subsequently sought a second round of public comment. No further comments were received concerning the proposed lower limit.

A limit on the amount of fluid that can be lost from thawed poultry was set to assist in preventing deceptive or misleading practices and not set for food safety reasons. For example, because poultry is purchased by weight, the presence of additional water would increase the final weight of the product meaning that consumers could be paying for water and not meat. Water may be used when poultry is processed to remove visible contamination and to chill the carcass. This will result in some water being absorbed by the poultry. The limit aims to recognise that while some water may be absorbed during processing, it should not be excessive.

Regulatory Problem

Following some recent surveillance of fluid loss from thawed poultry, the Australian poultry industry raised concerns that it may not be feasible to consistently comply with the current fluid loss limit of 6 per cent for thawed poultry. Industry has indicated this is mainly due to the implementation of Hazard Analysis Critical Control Programmes (HACCP) in the poultry processing sector in 1997 and a market preference for larger birds. HACCP has lead to an increase in the number of washing steps during processing, the volume and pressure of water used for washing and the need for poultry to spend longer in water chillers to achiever lower carcass temperatures. The market preference for larger birds has also meant longer times are needed to chill these birds.

Therefore the current 6 per cent limit may no longer be achieving its regulatory objective i.e. to ensure poultry processors minimise the uptake of water in poultry to be frozen, as industry has indicated it is having difficulty meeting this limit due to changes in its practices. Water uptake is also an issue for all poultry, not just frozen poultry. If fresh poultry were bulked with water, the limit would not apply.

Consultation

This issue arose just prior to the finalisation of the poultry Draft Assessment Report. While it is considered appropriate to address this issue within this report, stakeholder input needed to be sought, prior to the report's completion, to better inform the consultation process. This was achieved through the release of a discussion paper from 10 - 25 October 2005.

Summary of Submissions Received

Fifteen submissions were received in response to the discussion paper and a summary is provided at attachment 5.

Of the eight submissions received from industry, seven support increasing the limit to 8 per cent and calculating the limit over 20 birds to determine an average fluid loss. The remaining industry submission recognises that processors who use only water for chilling may have difficulty meeting the 6 per cent limit (this processor uses a combination of water and air chilling and therefore can meet the 6 per cent limit).

There were four government submissions from the Department of Health in Western Australia, Safe Food Production Queensland, Department of Human Services Victoria and the New Zealand Food Safety Authority. The Department of Health in WA supports retaining the 6 per cent limit but allowing it to be determined over a number of birds to determine an average fluid loss.

The Department of Health in WA also supports requiring poultry to be labelled with the percentage of water uptake. Safe Food Production Qld considers that this matter is best addressed through fair trading provisions and that the current limit is inappropriate given current processing technology. The Department of Human Services Victoria recognises that there may be a need to increase the limit for fluid loss for larger birds but recommends this issue be dealt with through HACCP Programmes and current practices. The New Zealand Food Safety Authority questions the need for the fluid loss limit in the Food Standards Code.

There was one submission from consumers, Australian Consumers Association (ACA). ACA does not believe there is sufficient justification to justify raising the level from 6 to 8 per cent and that more information should be obtained from New Zealand on whether New Zealand processors have difficulty meeting the 6 per cent limit.

The Food Technology Association of Victoria queried the justification to lower the level from 8 to 6 per cent during the review of the meat standard as it appears to have been made on the basis of one submission.

Worcestershire Scientific Services (United Kingdom) stated that this issue has caused much debate and analysis in Europe. A 6 per cent limit has been shown to be a workable ceiling for water uptake extraneous to the poultry by the European Commission (EC). This submitter also queried setting a limit on fluid loss as the issue relates to water uptake and chicken processors can use technologies to ensure water absorbed by chicken is retained. This water would therefore not be calculated as part of the fluid loss.

Summary of Data Received

Data was requested from government and industry on any testing conducted to assess compliance with the current 6 per cent limit. Raw data was received from the NSW Food Authority (results from testing on 4 frozen chickens), Department of Health in South Australia (results from testing on 2 frozen chickens) and from one major supermarket (results from testing on 38 frozen chickens). The Department of Health in WA and a poultry processor in New Zealand provided averaged results.

The results from raw data obtained from NSW, SA and the major supermarket indicated 68 per cent complied with the 6 per cent limit and 32 per cent did not. If an 8 per cent limit was in place, 89 per cent of the chickens would have complied and 11 per cent would not have.

The Department of Health in WA indicated the following:

- Of our two largest processors, water take up achieved by one processor is in the region 5.7 per cent for small birds and 4.9 per cent for large birds and the other processor is 5 per cent for all birds;
- Of a sample of 200 birds thawed annually by one processor, a fluid loss of 3.8 per cent (average) has been recorded; and
- Other processors' records show a 5 per cent (average fluid loss for thawed birds).

The processor from New Zealand, Tegel Foods stated that water pick up is measured routinely at some plants and at one of its plants, 900 samples were taken over a period of 3 months. The range was 1-14.9 per cent. This was measured by weighing and tagging birds pre-chill wash, recording the retention time in the chill wash, draining the birds for 20 minutes after chill wash and re-weighing them. The mean of the 900 samples was 5.5 per cent with a standard deviation of 2.26 per cent. This test only measured water pick up form the chill wash process – inevitably the birds would have picked up some water from the scalding, plucking, washing and evisceration before the pre-chill wash weighing. No data was available from the remaining jurisdictions, including New Zealand. While requested, no data was received from the poultry processors in Australia or other processors in New Zealand, with respect to results from testing fluid loss limits in frozen poultry.

International Regulations

European Union: Fluid loss limits apply to fresh, chilled or frozen whole carcasses as well as portions of poultry. Different limits apply depending on the method of chilling and the test method used. For frozen poultry that is chilled by immersion and tested using a drip test, a 5.1 per cent limit applies. This is determined as an average over 20 carcasses.

United States of America (USA)

Previously, the USA permitted 8-12 per cent fluid loss, 8 per cent for whole poultry and 12 per cent for poultry portions and ice packed poultry. In 1997, the USA Food Safety Inspection Service was taken to court on these limits (the Kenney case) and the USA District Court determined that the water absorption and retention limits were arbitrary and capricious because there was no demonstrated evidence for the basis of the limits. Since this ruling, processors must be able to justify (with data collected in accordance with a written protocol) that any water up-take is from meeting food safety requirements or time/temperature chilling requirements. If water up-take has not been minimised, the product may be considered adulterated. The maximum percentage of retained water must also be declared on the label, where applicable.

Relevant Issues

Issues that have arisen in submissions and as a result of discussions with stakeholders.

Do Current Requirements for Declaration of Water Apply?

One submitter indicated that the requirements for declaration of added water. The effect of this requirement is that water must be declared if it constitutes 5 per cent or more of the final food. If water is used for processing at the lowest level necessary to perform this processing function.

Is the Setting of a Fluid loss Limit an Appropriate Mechanism to Address this Issue?

Several submissions queried whether setting a fluid loss limit was the appropriate mechanism to address the issue of frozen poultry being bulked with excess water and suggested other ways this issue could be addressed.

If a Fluid loss Limit is set, should it just be for Frozen Poultry/Carcasses?

The current limit only applies to frozen poultry carcasses, which represents a very small percentage of the poultry market. For example, in the submission from Golden Cockerel it is indicated that frozen birds represent <1 per cent of current chicken production. The European Union sets limits for all poultry, frozen, fresh and portions. The US requirements apply to all meat, including poultry. If limits were set for fresh poultry, they would need to be calculated by weighing poultry post evisceration before immersion chilling and then post chilling, before being packed.

Can we justify continuing to regulate water uptake of frozen poultry, when there are no regulations that apply to the bulking of other meats or seafood with water?

Several submissions indicated that it was inconsistent to only set limits for poultry and not other meats.

The fluid loss limit for frozen chicken was included in the Code to recognise that when frozen chickens are thawed, fluid loss occurs. This fluid will consist of fluid that is normally present in chicken that is lost because of cellular breakdown during the thawing process but it may also contain water that has been absorbed during processing. The intent of the limit is to ensure that processors do not allow poultry to uptake water in excess of what is unavoidable during primary processing.

When other animals such as cattle, lambs and pigs are slaughtered, water is used to wash carcasses but is not used for chilling. There is therefore minimal, if any, uptake of water during the primary processing of these animals. Hence, there is no need for limits to be set. Water may be used when these meats are further processed would apply i.e. if water is used as an ingredient, it would need to be declared where it constitutes 5 per cent or more of the final food.

Water may be used to process seafood for washing and chilling. Different methods are used to cool seafood, depending on the type of seafood. Methods used include iced water, ice slurries and ice/salt slurries. Where water is used for chilling, the seafood could potentially absorb water during the cooling process.

The use of water during the processing of any animal, including seafood would be subject to the same requirements as that applying to poultry.

Should Different Limits be set For Different Sized Birds?

One submission from government indicated that a higher limit may be applicable for larger birds. Larger birds take longer to chill and therefore, if they are water chilled, they will be exposed to water longer than smaller birds and potentially uptake more water. Industry has not indicated that different limits should be set for different sized birds, but does support the limit being averaged over 20 birds so variabilities such as bird size, can be taken into account. If a fluid loss limit is stipulated, these variabilities need to be considered.

If an Average is Permitted, Should all Birds Tested be the Same Size or Varying Sizes?

One submission queried whether all the birds tested should be the same

size when the fluid loss limit is calculated over a number of birds. Industry has argued that the testing of fluid loss should be calculated over a number of birds, because variability will occur, particularly between different sized poultry.

Therefore, different sized poultry could be used to determine this average.

Should the Method of Analysis be Reviewed?

Many submissions supported changing the method of analysis to allow fluid loss to be calculated over a number of birds.

Maintain the Status Quo

This means the 6 per cent limit would be retained as well as the method of analysis. Poultry processors using water chilling have indicated they have difficulty meeting the 6 per cent limit due to:

- The introduction of HACCP (in 1997) requiring:

  – Additional washes and an increase in the volume and pressure of water used;

  – Additional chilling time to achieve lower carcass temperatures;

Industry has also indicated the method of analysis, by not allowing an average to be calculated over a number of birds, does not recognise the range in moisture uptake that occurs due to inherent variability in incoming flocks.

Industry has stated that if the current requirements are retained, food safety will be compromised to comply with the limits. Specifically, less contact time will occur in the chiller tanks. The chiller tanks lower carcass temperatures but also, provided free chlorine is available, can be effective at reducing microbial contamination of the carcass.

While industry has provided justification for increasing the limit to 8 per cent, data provided from the Department of Health in WA, where the current 6 per cent limit has been actively enforced, indicates poultry processors within this State can consistently meet the current limit, provided an average is calculated.

Regulatory Impact

It is unclear whether industry can meet the 6 per cent limit, without compromising food safety due to the contradiction between the information provided by industry and the Department of Health in WA. However, the information from the Department of Health in WA and industry suggests that the setting of an absolute limit may be unreasonable.

The regulatory impact of having to meet an absolute limit would be high if enforcement officers rigourously enforced the current fluid loss limit. Penalties would apply for any non-complying frozen birds. A greater impact would be supermarkets refusing to sell frozen poultry that was not in compliance. This was threatened when this issue arose and as poultry processor cannot always guarantee that frozen poultry will meet the 6 per cent limit, they may not be able to sell their product. Therefore not preferred due to the potential difficulty and associated costs industry may experience when trying to comply with an absolute limit.

Retain a Limit but Allow this Limit to be Calculated over an Average number of birds

There is conflicting evidence as to whether a 6 or 8 per cent limit is appropriate. Industry strongly favours applying an 8 per cent limit that is calculated as an average over 20 birds. However, the Department of Health in WA has indicated processors within this State can and do routinely meet the 6 per cent limit.

Therefore, if a limit is to be applied, further discussions with industry and government should occur as to what would be an appropriate limit. A limit should allow for the unavoidable water uptake that occurs during poultry processing but not be too high such that it effectively permits the absorption of water excess to processing needs. In particular, discussions should occur with poultry processors in WA who appear to be consistently meeting the 6 per cent limit, as to their views on this issue. While processors in New Zealand have had to comply with a 6 per cent limit since it was introduced in the 1970s, they have indicated they have difficulty consistently meeting this limit.

Therefore, while it is debateable as to whether a 6 or 8 per cent limit is appropriate, it seems reasonable to allow the limit to be calculated over a number of birds, to account for the variabilities that will occur. Allowing an average to be calculated was well supported in submissions.

Regulatory Impact

Allowing an average to be calculated would go someway to addressing industry. However, there is conflicting evidence as to what an appropriate limit might be. If a limit were applied to frozen birds, it would only address the issue of water uptake in these birds. This issue applies to all poultry. Therefore, as it does not fully address the regulatory problem of water uptake in all poultry, in excess of processing needs.

Delete the Requirement and Defer to Fair Trading/Food Act Offences

If the requirement were deleted and there was a concern that a poultry processor was allowing excessive water uptake to bulk product,

Recourse could be available through the:

- General offences under the State/Territory Food Acts which prohibit misleading or deceptive practices or sale of food not complying with purchaser's demands; or
- Fair trading legislation.

Several State jurisdictions in Australia support deleting the fluid loss limit and deferring the matter to fair trading legislation.

In respect to fair trading legislation, the ACCC has advised that if the fluid loss limit were deleted, there is nothing specific in State/Territory fair trading legislation that would stop processors from adding excess water. However, consumers could have a case for being misled if the label does not indicate that water has been 'added'. State/Territory fair trading legislation is not enforced unless there is a complaint from a consumer or business. There would also be no guidance for processors as to what would be considered misleading unless it was provided.

Having no requirement in relation to the unnecessary uptake of water in poultry may not provide adequate assurance for consumers,

For the following reasons:

- If some poultry is bulked with water, and there is no labelling to this affect, consumers may be misled as they will be unknowingly paying for water;
- There would be no enforcement of water uptake in poultry and therefore poultry processors may maximise rather than minimise water uptake; and
- Consumers concerned about water loss would need to make a complaint and in the absence of any guidance on what percentage of water uptake would be considered excessive, it may be difficult to assess whether this was occurring.

Regulatory Impact

The least costly for industry and government, as there would be no requirement to comply with or enforce. However, it offers the least assurance to consumers that water uptake is being minimised by poultry processors.

If a poultry processor allowed water absorption to occur, in excess of processing needs to improve profit margins, the consumer may unwittingly pay more for poultry than it should.

Delete Fluid loss Limit and Reinforce obligation to Minimise Water

The limit on fluid loss for frozen poultry could be deleted and poultry processors specifically referred to their legal obligations, with respect to the use of water as a processing aid. Where water is used to assist with processing (such as for the removal of visible contamination from carcasses and for chilling), it must be used at the lowest level necessary to perform this processing function. For example, during chilling, the contact time with the poultry should be the minimum necessary to achieve the required temperature. If water is used in excess of what is necessary to meet processing needs, it is not considered a 'processing aid' but an ingredient that is added to the food and must therefore be declared in accordance. Added water must be declared if it constitutes 5 per cent or more of the final food.

Poultry processors could be reminded of these legal obligations through the inclusion of an editorial note within the proposed Standard for poultry meat. As this Standard will only apply in Australia, the New Zealand Food Safety Authority has advised they would bring these obligations to the attention of their poultry processors through another mechanism. These obligations would be further explained in the interpretive guide for the Standard for Poultry Meat and would advise on appropriate practices to minimise water uptake and what would be considered to be a reasonable percentage of water uptake, having regard to bird size.

The objective of setting a fluid loss limit, which is to minimise water uptake in frozen poultry by reinforcing the current legal obligations on poultry processors to ensure water uptake does not exceed what is unavoidable during primary processing. While a fluid loss limit would indirectly require poultry processors to minimise water uptake, fluid loss in itself, is not the issue. The issue is excessive water uptake.

The editorial note would also clarify that the obligations apply to all poultry, not just frozen poultry. Water uptake is an issue for all poultry that is water chilled.

Regulatory Impact

There is no regulatory impact for either industry or government as it is a reinforcement of the current obligations.

As it will highlight poultry processors obligations with respect to minimising water uptake in all poultry. However, there may be a concern that in the absence of an actual legal limit, enforcement will be more difficult and therefore consumers may not be as adequately protected. To address this concern, the guidance provided in the interpretive guide needs to be clear on what steps poultry processors need to take to minimise water uptake and the percentage of water uptake that would be considered reasonable.

Require the Percentage of Water Uptake to be Declared on the Label

The discussion paper queried whether this issue could be addressed in other ways such as labelling poultry with the percentage of water content.

The Department of Health in Western Australia strongly supports the labelling of poultry with average percentage water content. However, it was not supported by industry. One industry submission stating that it is not practical or sensible to label carcasses with the percentage of water content. Industry submissions also queried its value to consumers with a New Zealand processor stating that as processors within New Zealand use similar processes, the percentage water content will be similar.

If labelling were required, it would be more meaningful for the percentage of water uptake to be declared. It would also need to be expressed as an average. Otherwise the percentage of water uptake for every poultry carcass would need to be determined and uniquely labelled, which would be very costly and impractical.

If an average were required to be included in the label, it is uncertain whether this would be effective in ensuring poultry processors minimise the amount of water absorbed by poultry during processing. It could provide an incentive to minimise water uptake, if a lower stated average percentage water pickup gave a poultry producer a competitive edge. For this to be effective, consumers would need to understand that the lower the stated percentage, the less retained water is present in the poultry and hence it represents better value for money.

Those poultry processors that exclusively use water for chilling as processors that use a combination of air and water or air only would have less water absorption occurring. The chicken meat industry has advised that approximately 75 per cent of chicken carcasses are chilled using water only, with the remainder being chilled using a combination of water and air and a very small percentage air only.

Regulatory Impact

The most expensive for industry as in addition to minimising water uptake during processing,

It would have to calculate the average percentage of water uptake occurring and Print this average in the label.

It could also unduly penalise those processors who exclusively use water for chilling, which for chicken meat sector is approximately 75 per cent of the market.

Benefit consumers if poultry could be compared, through the average percentage of water stated on the label, to determine which is the best value for money.

However, as indicated by a New Zealand processor, as the processes used are similar, the averages stated may also be similar.

The potential cost to processors, particularly those who use water for chilling. The benefit to consumers is also uncertain.

Conclusion and Recommendations

Standard for Poultry Meat: The Standard does not include retail, as the risk assessment concluded that the potential risks from poultry at the retail stage of the poultry meat supply chain are adequately addressed through current management systems. However, the risk assessment did identify consumers as an important contributor to the safety of poultry meat and although consumers cannot be covered under a standard, FSANZ proposes to work with the Poultry Cooperative Research Centre in developing a more targeted food safety education strategy to improve consumer handling of raw poultry.

Requirements at Primary Production

A businesses involved in the growing of poultry intended for sale for human consumption (and includes breeding, hatching and transporting to the processing facility) to systematically examine all of their operations to identify potential poultry food safety hazards and implement controls that are commensurate with the food safety risk. In particular, the controls must minimise contamination of poultry from –

(a) Breeder stock; and

(b) Wild and domestic animals and birds; and

(c) Insects and rodents; and

(d) Drinking water; and

(e) Feed and litter; and

(f) Personnel; and

(g) Equipment.

Requirements at Processing

- Develop and implement a HACCP based food safety management system as currently required under State/Territory legislation which mandates compliance with the Australian Standard for Construction of Premises and Hygienic Production of Poultry Meat for Human Consumption AS 4465:2001 (the Australian Standard);
- Be obligated to ensure farmers supplying them with poultry are minimising food safety hazards (to support the requirement on poultry primary production businesses); and
- Maintain sufficient records to enable poultry and poultry meat products to be traced, where necessary for food safety.

Statement of Reasons

A Standard for Poultry Meat specifying requirements at the primary production and processing stages of the poultry meat supply chain of the Code for the following reasons:

- The proposed variation to the Code is consistent of the FSANZ Act to reduce the incidence of food-borne illness in Australia through a whole-of-chain approach to the safety of poultry;
- At the primary production stage, the new requirement for poultry farming operations to control their food safety hazards will address the residual risk identified by the scientific assessment, with the aim of lowering the percentage of poultry contaminated with Salmonella and Campylobacter spp;
- At the processing stage, although the scientific assessment did not identify a residual risk/no gaps in current strategies, the transfer of the current food safety requirements for poultry processing within State/Territory legislation to a Standard for Poultry Meat, will enable a whole-of-chain approach to the safety of poultry within the Code;
- The new legal requirements proposed for poultry farming operations and processors strengthen existing arrangements between processors and poultry farmers that supply processors, by enabling enforcement agencies to scrutinise these existing arrangements and to intervene where necessary; and
- The cost-benefit analysis is the most cost effective means of addressing the food safety hazards within the poultry meat supply chain.

Other Poultry Requirements in the Code

Two existing requirements within the Code that apply to poultry were evaluated as part of this proposal.

Eviscerated Poultry

Statement of Reasons: Processing Requirements be deleted for the following reasons:

- It permits poultry to be sold that is not completely eviscerated which is in conflict with the Australian Standard which requires poultry to be completely eviscerated and is currently mandatory under State and Territory legislation; and
- Partly eviscerated poultry has the potential to be highly contaminated with pathogenic bacteria and therefore poses an unacceptable risk to consumers.

Limit on Fluid Loss from Thawed Poultry

During the development of the standard, the Australian poultry industry raised concerns that it may not be feasible to consistently meet the current legal limit applying to fluid loss from frozen whole birds. The current fluid loss limit in the Code is 60 g/kg (6 per cent) of thawed poultry and was set in 2000 as part of the process of developing a meat standard for the joint Australia New Zealand Food Standards Code. Prior to this, the limit for fluid loss was 80 g/kg (8 per cent) in Australia and 60 g/kg in New Zealand. The Australian poultry industry has indicated a preference for returning to the 8 per cent limit. A limit is set in the Code to prevent fraudulent practices i.e. to prevent the bulking of frozen poultry with water.

MODERN MEAT CHICKEN INDUSTRY

The modern broiler industry has developed a hybrid that is unlike any other breed. The initial breeds used in modern broiler hybrids were Cornish and Plymouth Rocks. Today's broiler can achieve a 5-pound market weight in five weeks. Forty years ago, it took 10 weeks to achieve a 4-pound market weight. These advances are the result of scientific progress in genetic, nutritional, and environmental research.

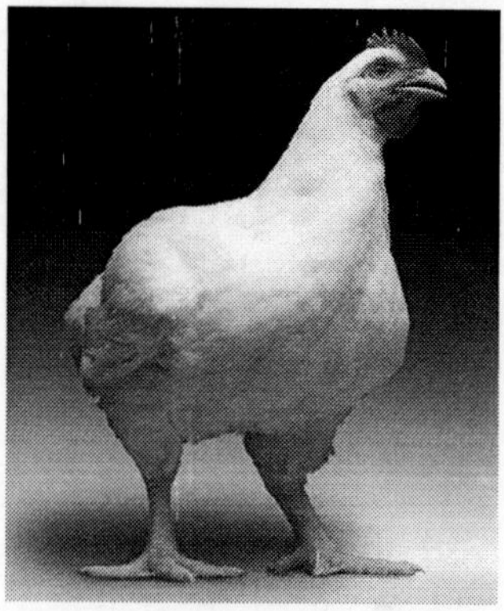

Primary Breeders

The primary breeder flocks are owned by an international breeder company. These flocks produce highly efficient breeding lines (parent lines) that are sold to the integrated broiler companies. Chicks are hatched at the breeder's hatchery and then sold and delivered to the integrated companies' parent breeding farms.

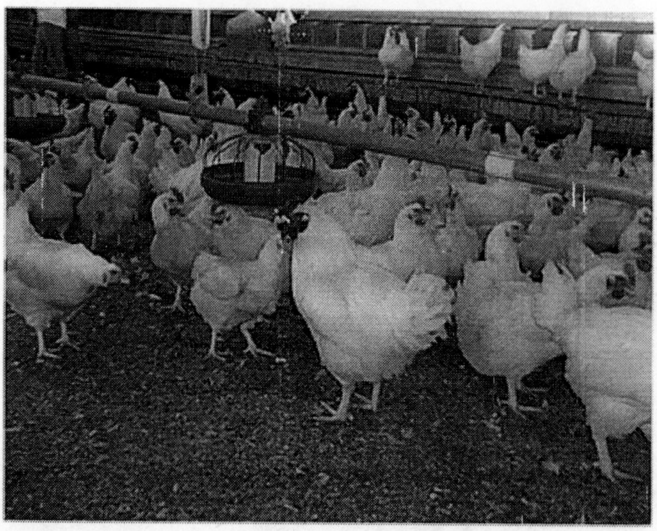

Parent Stock Breeders

Once the chicks arrive at the integrated company's breeder growing farm, the birds are raised to 20 weeks of age under environmentally controlled conditions. Controlling the length of daylight is extremely important. Breeders do not receive more than 10 hours of light daily as they are growing so they are not prematurely stimulated to lay eggs. During the 20 weeks of the grow- out, each bird will eat 30-35 pounds of feed and will grow to 6-8 lbs. Once they reach 20 weeks of age, they are transported to the breeder farm.

The parent breeders are the birds that produce the fertile eggs that will become the broiler chickens that are harvested for meat. Breeders are raised in open floor houses with automatic watering, feeding, and egg collection systems. Males and females are allowed to mate naturally. Females begin producing eggs around 24 weeks of age and will lay efficiently for 40 weeks per cycle. An average broiler breeder female will lay 150-180 eggs in a year.

Hatching Eggs

When the broiler breeder female reaches 24 weeks of age, she will be laying. It takes a female between 24 and 32 hours to produce a fertile egg.

The eggs are automatically collected daily, transported to the hatchery, and stored at 55-65° F and 70 per cent humidity until they are set in the incubator. The eggs are held here for about three to 10 days prior to being placed in an incubator. One fertile hatching egg is worth $.28 each and weighs around 65g.

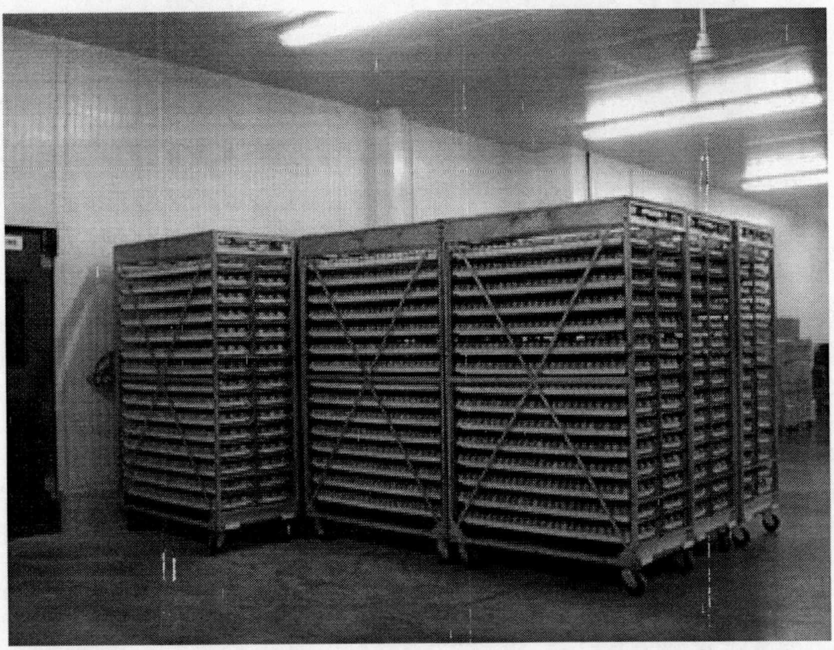

Incubation

Most Integrated companies own their own hatchery to produce the chicks. Incubators will hold thousands e eggs in a very controlled environment. They are then transferred into hatching baskets. On the 21st day the chicks hatch.

Hatching

After the chicks hatch, they are removed from the hatchers and processed before being taken to the grow-out farm. Processing of broiler chickens include sexing (separating the males and females if the company raised the two sexes separately) and vaccination. They are then counted and placed in baskets for delivery to the farm within 12 hours of hatch. A broiler chick is worth about $.36 and weights around 44g.

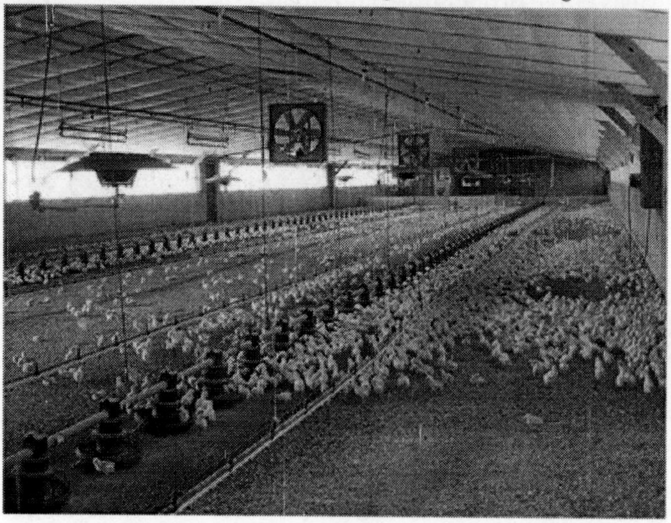

Grow-out

The chicks are then placed in floor rearing houses where they are raised under environmentally controlled conditions. Ventilation of the broiler house is criti.cal for controlling temperature and humidity in the grow-out house.

Birds are grown to different sizes depending on the market they are meant to fill. On average a broiler consumes about 9 pounds of feed (current cost of about $1.50 or $.30/pound) and reaches 5 pounds (live weight) in 5 weeks.

When the birds reach the desired weight, a company catching crew will catch and load the birds onto trucks to be transported to the processing plant. The catching crew takes a great deal of care in carefully handling the birds to prevent bruises or injury.

Harvesting

At the processing plant, birds are humanely slaughtered as quickly as possible. After slaughter, the feathers, offal , head, legs, and other items are removed so that they have a whole dressed carcass ready for sale or to send onto further processing.

The cost of processing a broiler is about $.18 per pound. The wholesale price for a whole broiler is about $.53 per pound.

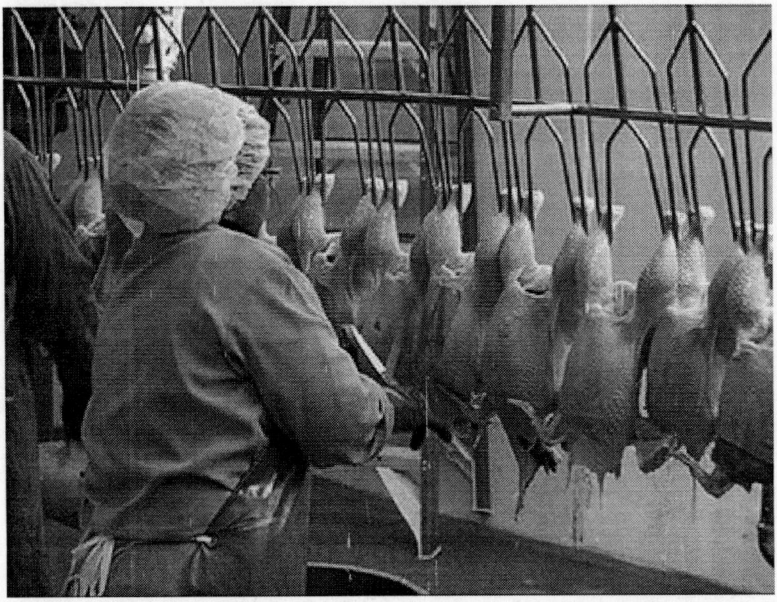

Further Processed Products

This is where we make the product more convenient as well as add value to the product. In the meat industry, further processing means something is done to the whole carcass such as cut-up, deboning, and fabricating poultry meat into value-added products. The cut-up operation is often done at the processing plant. However, some companies ship the whole carcasses to the further processing plant for specialized cut-up. Cut-up is where machines cut the whole carcass into individual parts. Deboning is where the bones are removed from specific parts to produce items like breast filets or other boneless products.

Value added refers to fabricating the carcass into consumer-ready products that requires additional time or labour. These products usually involve seasoning, breading, sauces, and marinating, as well as special packaging to meet market demands for convenient products. The added value result in higher margins and profits while providing a large product choice for the consumer.

□

6

The H5N1 Avian Influenza Virus

INTRODUCTION

The avian flu is a current and significant issue involving the global environment as well as the health of millions of people around the world. In the past few months, the imminent threat of an avian flu pandemic had drawn increasing public attention. This is due to the rapid spread of the virus among birds and to humans as well. In order to better battle the virus, we must develop a deeper understanding of how the avian flu works, where is comes from and how it affects the global environment as well the health of animals and humans.

The threat of the H5N1 avian influenza virus has been speculated to begin within the Guangdong Province deep within China; it has been known to be the "birthplace of the flu." This is because it is an area where animals and humans live in close proximity to each other for thousands of years, thus providing more opportunities for a virus to jump from animals to humans. This environmental factor becomes a dangerous living arrangement when it comes to the issue of the spread of diseases, such as the H5N1 influenza. Sadly, the story of the H5N1 avian influenza only begins there; it has spread to multiple continents and may be on the verge of becoming a global epidemic. So far, the hardest hit country is Vietnam. With multiple environmental, social, and ecological factors that promote the propagation of the virus, the country itself has become a microcosm of the impending pandemic of this new type of influenza among humans.

With a focus on the multiple factors that aid in the spread of the avian influenza in Vietnam, as well as other global environmental factors, we can strengthen our comprehension of the patterns of distribution of the virus as well as the environmental and physicochemical components that help promote and propagate it. By furthering the knowledge of these factors, we can better determine how to implement systems in which to contain the virus and treat the victims of the influenza. Therefore, this chapter will address the different environmental, ecological, and social factors within Vietnam as well as globally that has made it a prime breeding ground for the H5N1 virus and its advancement.

Others topics to be discussed will include: a study of another emerging virus that may prove to be a model for the H5N1 virus, an overview of the H5N1 avian influenza virus, the environmental circumstances that lead to the emergence and acceleration of the disease, the human transmission of the H5N1 avian influenza virus, environmental factors that lead to the spread of the virus within Vietnam and globally, and possible prevention policies.

Model for the H5n1 Avian Influenza Virus, West Nile

The spread and transmission of the West Nile virus can be used as prime example of how the environment plays a major part in the acceleration and progression of a virus both locally and globally. It is a virus that has many similarities in relation to the H5N1 virus. One similarity is that it is a virus that spreads through the use of a vector, in the case of the West Nile virus, it is mosquitoes, in the case of the H5N1 virus, it is birds. Another similarity in between these viruses is the condition that both viruses cannot be spread by human to human transmission. Through these factors, both environmental and man-made, the West Nile virus has made its way from the far regions of its origins into urban areas all over the world.

The West Nile virus was first reported in Uganda in 1937, even in today's world it is still most commonly found in Africa, West Asia, Europe, and the Middle East. In the summer of 1999, the West Nile virus surprised scientists and was found North America, more specifically in New York City. Since its first appearance in New York City, it has been seen in birds and mosquitoes in every state in the United States except Alaska and Hawaii. West Nile virus has now been named a seasonal endemic within the United States.

The West Nile virus is a mosquito-borne virus that can cause a wide range of symptoms with varying severity in humans. The most fatal consequence of contracting the West Nile virus is encephalitis, the inflammation of the brain, the membranes surrounding the brain and the spinal cord. Other serious symptoms of the virus include fever, stupor, neck stiffness, disorientation, coma, tremors, convulsions, muscle weakness, vision loss, numbness, and paralysis. Some of these symptoms are temporary; however the neurological symptoms may become permanent.

Individuals of all ages are susceptible to this virus through mosquitoes; however the West Nile virus proves to be more of a danger to the elderly and young children in terms of the severity of the symptoms and the permanent damage that it may cause.

Natural environmental conditions and factors that led to the spread of the West Nile virus all the way to North America include local conditions such as the multiple sites and locations which prove to be advantageous to the proliferation of the vector of the virus, the mosquitoes. Another environmental factor that led to the spread of the West Nile virus to North America is global warming. In combination with other man-made environmental factors, the spread of the West Nile virus in North America was made possible by these local as well as global natural environmental factors.

Local natural environmental factors within New York City made the location advantageous for the West Nile virus to become endemic to the city during the summers. In a concentrated urban location such as the city, there are various places in which stagnant water will collect throughout the area after a rainfall. These accumulations of stagnant water make them a choice location for the breeding of mosquitoes, which may carry the West Nile virus.

Global warming is also an enormous contributor the expansion of the West Nile virus to North America. It is global warming that has provided North America with unusually high temperatures during the summer months which allow for the vectors of West Nile virus to thrive in an area that they would not normally live for long. The warmer temperatures in New York City due to global warming permitted mosquitoes to breed and infect the local bird population as well as humans.

In addition to the natural environmental factors that provided optimal conditions for the West Nile virus to expand, there are also local and global man-made environmental factors that allow for the continuing advancement of the West Nile virus. One of the local man-made environmental factors is the dense population over a small location, which is characteristic of most cities, especially New York City. A global environmental factor that affects the travel of this virus is the transport of animals that may carry the West Nile virus. Both man-made environmental factors have made a tremendous impact on the speed and range of distribution of the propagation of the virus.

Local man-made environmental factors such as the concentrated amount of people over a small space provide the opportunity of mosquitoes that carry the West Nile virus to infect more people over its short life span. Another man-made environmental factor that contributes to the rise in population of mosquitoes is the multiple products that can collect rainwater and become a makeshift habitat for the breeding of mosquitoes. Some of these products include, bird baths, junk yards, and many others that can collect rainfall.

Global travel of animals can lead to the inadvertent movement of viruses. There are multiple animals which can be infected with the West Nile virus, some of which include birds, pigs, dogs, cats, and sometimes horses. These animals may be transported to other locations and a non-infected mosquito may bite infected animals and then transfer the virus to other animals in an area that had no previous occurrence of the virus. Therefore, transported animals can perpetuate a cycle in which the virus is transferred from mosquito to animals and to possibly humans. With the propagation of the virus in other animals, the virus can move quickly to other areas in this way.

By observing the many factors that contribute to the spread of the West Nile virus, it can also allow for further insights into how the H5N1 avian influenza virus may possibly spread and travel across the world as well. The West Nile virus supplies a model in which, according to the similarities between the West Nile virus and the H5N1 avian influenza virus may show scientists how to better estimate the pathways of distribution of the virus. The H5N1 avian influenza virus is an absolutely separate entity from any other known virus; however by studying the patterns of similar viruses, it can provide scientists insight into the possible scenarios that may occur.

The H5n1 Avian Influenza Virus

Influenza A (H5N1) virus, also called H5N1 virus, is an influenza A virus subtype that occurs mainly in birds, is highly contagious among birds, and can be deadly to them. The avian influenza is an infection caused by viruses that naturally occurs among birds. The virus is contagious among multiple types of birds and can make some domesticated birds; including chickens, ducks, and turkeys, very sick and can potentially kill them.

Vulnerable birds become infected when they come in contact with contaminated secretions or with surfaces that are contaminated with secretions from infected birds. The infection of avian influenza viruses in domestic poultry causes two main forms of the disease that are distinguished by low and high extremes of virulence. The highly pathogenic form spreads more rapidly through flocks of poultry. This form may cause diseases that affects multiple internal organs and has a mortality rate that can reach 90 to a 100 per cent often within 48 hours.

Outbreaks of avian influenza H5N1 occurred among poultry in eight countries in Asia during late 2003 and early 2004. These countries are Cambodia, China, Indonesia, Japan, Laos, South Korea, Thailand, and Vietnam. At that time, more than 100 million birds in the affected countries either died from the disease or were killed in order to try to control the outbreaks. By March 2004, the outbreaks were reported to be under control due to the large groups of domesticated poultry as well as wild birds being destroyed.

Since late June 2004, however, new outbreaks of influenza H5N1 among poultry were reported by several countries in Asia and Europe. These countries are Cambodia, China, Indonesia, Kazakhstan, Malaysia, Mongolia, Russia, Thailand, and Vietnam. The H5N1 avian influenza virus infection also has been reported among poultry in Turkey and Romania and among wild migratory birds in Croatia. Human cases of H5N1 avian influenza virus infection have been reported in Cambodia, China, Indonesia, Thailand, and Vietnam. The country of Vietnam is being hit the most heavily with human and animal deaths due to natural and man-made ecological and environmental factors that help the virus proliferate within their communities.

Human Transmission

The avian influenza is very species-specific, but in rare cases has been known to cross the species barrier and affect humans. During an outbreak of avian influenza among poultry, there is a possible risk to people who have contact with infected birds or surfaces that have been contaminated with secretions from infected birds. Symptoms of avian influenza in humans have ranged from typical human influenza-like symptoms and other severe and life-threatening complications. There are only three known subtypes of influenza A viruses, which are the H1N1, H1N2, and H3N2 viruses currently circulating among humans. It is likely that some genetic parts of current human influenza A viruses came from birds originally. Influenza A viruses are constantly changing, and they might adapt over time to infect and spread among humans.

One of the first instances of the H5N1 influenza outbreak among humans was in Hong Kong in 1997; Dr. Margaret Chan was the city's director of health at the time. At the confirmation that it was the H5N1 virus, she ordered the eradication of the disease's presumable host, 1.4 million ducks and chickens within the city, thus causing the temporary withdrawal of the disease. The disease killed six people of eighteen individuals with documented clinical cases of the virus.

The risk from avian influenza is generally low to most people because the viruses occur mainly among birds and do not usually infect humans. However, more than 100 human cases of avian influenza infection have been reported since 1997. Most cases of avian influenza infection in humans have resulted from contact with infected poultry or surfaces contaminated with secretions from infected birds. The spread of avian influenza viruses from one ill person to another has been reported very rarely, and transmission has not been observed to continue beyond one person.

Of the few avian influenza viruses that have crossed the species barrier to infect humans, H5N1 has caused the largest number of detected cases of severe disease and death in humans. In the current outbreaks in Asia and Europe, more than half of those infected with the virus have died. Most cases have occurred in previously healthy children and young adults. However, it is possible that the only cases currently being reported are those in the most severely ill people, and that the full range of illnesses caused by the H5N1 virus has not yet been defined.

So far, the spread of H5N1 virus from person to person has been rare and has not continued beyond one person. Nonetheless, because all influenza viruses have the ability to mutate, scientists are concerned that the H5N1 virus could be able to infect humans and spread easily from one person to another. Because these viruses do not commonly infect humans, there is little or no immune protection against them in the human population. If the H5N1 virus were to gain the capacity to spread easily from person to person, an influenza pandemic otherwise known as a worldwide outbreak of disease could begin. No one can predict when a pandemic might occur. However, experts from around the world are watching the H5N1 avian influenza virus situation in Asia and Europe very closely and are preparing for the possibility that the virus may begin to spread more easily and widely from person to person.

H5N1 Avian Influenza, the Physicochemical Components of the Virus

The H5N1 avian influenza virus is barely one-thousandth of a millimeter; it has to be magnified 200,000 times in order to be seen on an electron microscope. This incredibly small life-form can potentially be the cause of a pandemic that in theory; could be the greatest killer in human history. This virus could conceivably take the lives of millions, even hundreds of millions of people all around the world. The increased understanding of how physicochemical factors affect the propagation of this virus might provide insight which can be useful in determining a policy in order to prevent or at the very least stall the pandemic.

In order for a virus to become a full blown pandemic, it has to fulfill three conditions outlined by the World Health Organization. The first prerequisite being that it has to be an entirely new strain of virus that is unknown to humans for more than a century. The next qualification is that the virus has been proven to jump species. And finally the last stipulation that constitutes the definition of a pandemic is known instances of the virus being transmitted easily and freely from human to human. So far, the H5N1 avian influenza virus has completed two of the three provisions.

In dealing with the first provision, the H5N1 virus is an absolutely new strain of virus that is not known to humans. This virus, until the past decade has been known to affect birds only and at different intensities. The fact that it is unknown to humans for more than a century means that no human is immune to the virus. Without prior knowledge of the virus, the human body is not equipped to attack the virus and prevent it from ravaging the body and its systems.

Since it is an entirely unknown virus to the human body, the H5N1 avian influenza virus is a dangerous virus that can cause many potentially fatal secondary symptoms within the body. The virus works by entering the body and invading an individual cell. Within the cell, the virus will essentially seize the cell's life materials and replicates itself at a rapid rate. When the virus and its multiple copies break out of the now dead cell, it will continue to invade various cells of the body, thus killing the cells. By doing so, the virus will cause fluid to flood the lungs. The affected individual will either die by basically drowning in their own fluids or of many other secondary problems, which range from fever, cough, sore throat, and muscle aches to eye infections, pneumonia, severe respiratory diseases, the least of which include acute respiratory distress. In reported cases of individuals affected with the H5N1 virus, it can be clearly seen that the virus has successfully accomplished the first condition necessary to become a pandemic.

The second condition that must be fulfilled by the H5N1 virus is the ability to jump from species to species. There have been various instances of the avian virus found in multiple species of animals. There have been cases where the avian influenza virus was present in dogs, cats, and pigs. The most notable case however was in 2004; when the avian influenza virus killed 147 Bengal tigers in a Thailand zoo. Scientists are still determining if theses cases of avian influenza in other animals can also cause spread to humans, but as so far, the only method in which to contract the avian influenza virus is still through direct contact with infected poultry or contact with secretions of infected poultry. The instance of the presence of the H5N1 influenza virus among different species demonstrates the accelerated evolution of the virus itself.

The H5N1 avian influenza virus has been described by many scientists as a sloppy, capricious and promiscuous virus. The H5N1 virus, once it has entered a living cell can produce 100,000 copies of itself within an hour, with each succeeding copy making another 100,000 copies. At such a breakneck speed of breeding, the virus will most certainly make mistakes in its copying and end up with various mutations. It then becomes possible that one of these mutations will have the right combination which allows it to travel easily from human to human. The H5N1 virus, with its quick advancement in terms of evolution, has allowed it to satisfy the second prerequisite for a potential pandemic.

The final and third qualification for defining a pandemic has not yet been fulfilled by the H5N1 virus. Despite its quick evolutionary rate, the avian influenza virus has yet been able to be easily transmitted from person to person. There have been cases in which humans have passed the virus to one another, but not yet easily and regularly. Once this final condition has been met the H5N1 virus, it will become a full blown pandemic that the world is not prepared for.

There are two ways in which scientists speculate that the H5N1 virus will be able to make the jump into the third condition. One possibility is that since the evolutionary rate of the virus is so accelerated and careless, the virus will on its own, stumble across a mutation that will have the correct combination that will allow it to be transmitted from human to human. The other possibility, the more likely one according to world scientists, is that the H5N1 virus will infect an individual who already has the human influenza virus. By doing so, the H5N1 virus could exchange genes with the human virus and therefore become easy to pass on. Whichever way the H5N1 virus chooses to cross the threshold into becoming a pandemic, it has become only a matter of time.

The Environmental Factors Within Vietnam

Within the microcosm of the country of Vietnam, the people have been hit with the virus most heavily, so much so that the World Health Organization has called it an endemic within the nation. It can be seen that numerous environmental factors play an imperative role in the promotion of the H5N1 avian influenza virus among humans. By examining how such environmental factors in Vietnam are aiding in the spread of the disease among animals and humans, the world can be able to battle the virus more competently.

One of the major environmental factors that has become a main issue is that of the living arrangements between animals and humans. In the Southeast Asia, more specifically the country of Vietnam, the majority of people reside in rural areas and make their livelihood by sustenance farming or live in crowded city areas. It is in situations like those in which the greater number of Vietnamese citizens live that provide a choice environment for the H5N1 virus to thrive.

In both the big cities and the small rural villages alike, animals such as poultry are in close quarters with their owners. For the citizens of Vietnam, the raising of animals such as poultry is a large part of their family income, which makes it an important part of their daily lives. In some cases, the animals share sleeping quarters with their owners. These types of living situations bring about optimal transmission of the H5N1 avian influenza virus from animals to humans. In other cases, seen throughout the country, mostly in the urban areas, there is just simply not enough living space to keep animals and people separate. By combining the living areas of both animals and the general population, infections of the virus become more likely to spread to humans.

The Main Global Environmental Factors

There are different environmental factors that affect the H5N1 avian influenza virus in various parts of the globe. However, there are two major environmental and ecological factors that span the entire world and are becoming large players in relation to the spread of the H5N1 virus among birds internationally and soon; when the virus fulfills the third condition of a pandemic, a major health issue for humans as well. For the time being, the H5N1 avian influenza virus remains easily transmitted among birds only. The seasonal migration of birds can allow for the spread of the disease from continent to continent. An instance in which migration of birds has caused the spread of the disease is in the case in which 5,000 birds, primarily bar-headed geese died of an H5N1 influenza infection in western China in the vicinity of the two-mile high Qinghai Lake in August of 2005. More than 100,000 rare birds and 189 types of avian species including the bar-headed geese migrate to and from Qinghai Lake each year. These birds migrate in a crisscross pattern that will lead as far as Europe, Australia and America.

The migratory patterns of different birds are interconnected and will at some point in time cross each other, which will permit the virus to be transferred to another group of birds heading to another part of the world, thus spreading the H5N1 avian influenza virus to all the corners of the world. In some cases, the migratory birds are silent carriers of the virus, exhibiting none of the symptoms characteristic of the H5N1 avian influenza virus. In this way, the birds are carrying this potentially deadly disease from one point to another and spreading it to other birds along the way.

Currently, the virus has migrated from China to Russia and infected poultry in Siberia. The same thing has happened in Kazakhstan, Mongolia, and Tibet. From there, the virus has moved relentlessly, infecting chickens and wild birds to the west in Chelyabinsk, a city in the Ural Mountains, which is the final geographic barrier between Asia and Europe. In the northern hemisphere, it has reached as close as Canada, and will soon reach Africa. The rapid appearance of the virus in such different and distant regions has caused alarm throughout the international community. Environmental factors such as the migratory patterns of wild birds throughout the world are being considered closely. It may provide scientists with an outlook in which to better determine where the virus will appear next. This may aid in their attempt to be prepared for the spread of the virus and their attempts to contain it.

The other major global environmental issue that plays a large role in the advancement of the H5N1 avian influenza virus is globalization. Globalization can be defined as the increasing integration of countries. It is a term that is mostly applied to the economic integration of countries around the world. In this case, globalization is used to describe the integration of countries around the world in terms of the ease in which individuals from any country can travel to different areas of another country. Through globalization, the progression of the H5N1 avian influenza virus may move through the world at a pace faster than scientists can anticipate, and also in which technology and research cannot possibly keep up with. Globalization will give the H5N1 avian influenza virus an opportunity to travel to various parts of the world without impediment.

One of the main concerns involving the spread of the H5N1 avian influenza virus and globalization is how human to human contraction is going to be affected once the virus has gained the ability to spread easily from human to human. Once it has developed the ability to spread easily from human to human, the major concern becomes the travel of individuals around the world, particularly air travel. Through air travel, an infected individual could infect dozens of people during their movement, those newly infected individuals would in turn, infect dozens more, and so on and so forth. Despite modern commercial aircrafts having filtration programmes that limit the chance of a passenger transmitting the disease farther then a few rows, air travel still presents a larger problem in the progression of the disease. In one day, flying from a city such as Hong Kong, travelers could carry the virus to every corner of the world, infecting people in airports, hotels and other crowded places. Globalization will be a monumental factor in the spread of the H5N1 avian influenza virus when it is able to be easily transmitted from human to human.

Possible Prevention Policies

The international community has been frantically attempting to develop plans and contingencies to prevent or stall the advancement of the H5N1 avian influenza virus. Currently, there is no commercially available vaccine to protect humans against the H5N1 virus that is being seen in Asia and Europe. However, vaccine development efforts are taking place. Another course of action being evaluated is plan of distribution of a vaccine to both animals as well as humans when an effective vaccine is developed.

The issue of developing an effective vaccine for both animals and humans is posing to be a difficult task for scientists. This is due to the rapid physicochemical changes the virus undergoes in a relatively short time period. Thus causing the virus to mutate faster and become resistant quicker to any of the vaccines that can be developed.

In dealing with developing a vaccine for birds in order to prevent further infection of birds around the world, that problem has probably been more difficult for the scientists than creating a human vaccine for the H5N1 avian influenza virus. This is due in majority to the actions taken by the Chinese government in attempting to prevent the spread of the virus to otherwise healthy, viable poultry. Their measures included injecting healthy chickens with a combination of medications, including a human antiviral medicine and amantadine, which is an antiviral medication used to treat influenza A. By vaccinating their poultry in this manner, the Chinese government essentially gave the H5N1 avian influenza virus an opportunity to develop a new strain of itself that is resistant to those medications.

In late August of 2005, the United States announced that it has successfully tested a vaccine for humans, which drew a worldwide sigh of relief. But as soon as the success of the vaccine was broadcasted, so were the doubts of its competency. Questions arose debating the effectiveness of the vaccine, with scientists speculating that the vaccine could be deemed useless due to the virus already having mutated to a different form, resistant to the vaccine. So far, there is only one known medication that is somewhat effective in treating human cases of the H5N1 avian influenza virus, which is called Tamiflu. Tamiflu is not a vaccine for the H5N1 virus; however it is an expensive antiviral medication that has a limited effectiveness against the H5N1 virus. Despite the limited effectiveness of Tamiflu, another problem of this medication is that there has been such a demand for it that there is no way to know if enough of the antiviral will be made in time to stall the pandemic.

The synthesis of an effective vaccine is one issue, but the prompt production of such a vaccine is another topic entirely. The mass production of a vaccine internationally proves to be a daunting challenge for pharmaceutical companies. Another dilemma would be the cost of production of the vaccine. It would not be possible for third world countries such as Vietnam to afford enough vaccine for the population of the entire nation.

Another point of contention with the plans for the prevention of a pandemic is the ability of distribution of an effective vaccine to the individuals of the world that are most susceptible to the H5N1 avian influenza virus. Computer modelers have devised rapid-action containment plans that are operative if implemented within 48 hours of the reported outbreak. The problem with these rapid-action containment plans is that they do not take into account the accessibility of the location of each outbreak. For instance, if an outbreak occurred in rural Vietnam, the containment plan could not be implemented due to the lack of paved roads in order for the authorities to arrive to the area within the time frame allotted. Therefore, despite the best intentions of computer modelers, reality does not work in their favour.

With the potential onslaught of the H5N1 avian influenza virus on the human population, the impact on multiple factors of life is going to be countless. This virus is speculated to be more destructive than the great influenza pandemic of 1918, which killed 50 million to 100 million people in a world that is one-third as populated as it is today. The transmission of this virus from person to person will have severe consequences for the world's political, economic, and almost all other aspects of life for humans.

When the H5N1 avian influenza virus steps into the realm of being a full- fledged pandemic, the implications would be limitless in terms of how the different facets of human life would be changed. Literally tens of millions of people, if not more people would die from this illness. Politically, it could completely change the international landscape in many ways.

There would be chaos, Third World regimes would fall, armies would be brought to their knees, security and police forces would flounder at a loss of what to do. Government officials would stand helpless, powerless to help their constituents. Economically, retail sales would plummet, stock and housing markets would collapse. Everywhere in the world, bodies would stack up unburied and hospitals would be filled beyond capacity with the dead and dying. Many scientists agree that this pandemic is imminent and the issue is not if, but when the H5N1 avian influenza virus will be able to be easily transmitted from person to person.

The attempts made by the World Health Organization have been providing a stall in the spread of the virus for the past few months. However, with the seasons changing and the birds of the world beginning their migration around the globe, the H5N1 avian influenza virus cannot be held back any longer. Their efforts in trying to evaluate and monitor the progress of this virus have met many obstacles. For example, the Chinese government has been obstructing the progress of World Health Organization officials in tracking the virus within the country. In addition to that, the Chinese government has also been concealing the number of outbreaks and reported human infections from the international community.

Besides political bureaucracy, there have been other factors that have stilted the World Health Organization's venture to determine the trajectory of the H5N1 avian influenza virus; social factors have played a role in creating barriers. For instance, cultural clashes between Vietnamese farmers and Western virologists are immense. In Vietnam, autopsies violate religious beliefs, and possibly infected H5N1 virus victims are often cremated before samples can be taken, thus causing major hurdles in tracking the disease's movement and progression.

The environmental considerations and implications of this virus can be devastating to the animal population around the world. Although this virus is currently only predominant in birds it has been known to spread to other animals. Some of the species that have been reported to be affected by the H5N1 avian influenza virus so far, besides wild and domesticated birds, have been pigs, dogs, and cats. If the H5N1 influenza virus can make the final jump into humans, it is possible that it could also make the jump to affect a majority of the world's mammals. This would most likely include domesticated animals and livestock, which could possibly increase the human rate of infection.

Another environmental issue that needs to be taken into account would be the large-scale decimation of the world's domesticated poultry population. Since the outbreak of this virus, governments have been ordering the mass elimination of the source, millions of chickens and ducks. The continued eradication of the domesticated bird population may lead to serious environmental, not to mention economical consequences. This proves to be an illogical approach to controlling the outbreaks and spread of the H5N1 virus. In the majority of the countries affected most heavily by this disease, such as Vietnam, the livelihood of their citizens depends on their domesticated poultry. The mass decimation of domesticated poultry would be the same as destroying and possibly ending the lives of the individuals in danger of the virus themselves. The decimation is not a possible solution in terms of controlling the outbreaks as well as in the humanitarian sense. It is unreasonable to ask the people of third world countries to bury their food, which is essentially what we are asking of them if we choose to decimate large masses of domesticated poultry.

Finally, the H5N1 avian influenza virus is an unavoidable threat that affects the international community, not only in terms of the human race, but the world's animal population as well. The physicochemical factors as well as environmental factors have allowed this virus to become an impending danger. As seen in the country of Vietnam, where the people have been hit the hardest, there seems to be no stopping of this pandemic. With Vietnam being used as a microcosm of what is to come, there are too many obstacles in which scientists must overcome, some of which include bureaucracy issues, cultural and social clashes, and many others.

As of recent weeks, the number of confirmed human deaths from the H5N1 avian influenza virus has rose to 135 confirmed cases of infection and of those cases, 69 deaths due to the virus. It can be clearly seen that this virus is not something that will go away and it demands the attention of not only international scientists, but the leaders of the world as well. It is only with the full cooperation on the parts of the governments of the world, and also the allied forces of the world's scientists and environmentalists that a plan may be devised in which to alleviate the effects of this imminent pandemic and hopefully, lessen the severity of the virus' impact on the human and animal populations.

Table: Cumulative Number of Confirmed Human Cases of Avian Influenza A (H5N1) Reported to World Health Organization since December 7, 2005

Date of onset	Cambodia		China		Indonesia		Thailand		Viet Nam		Total	
	cases	deaths	cases	deaths	cases	deaths	cases	deaths	cases	deaths	cases	deaths
26.12.03 - 10.03.04	0	0	0	0	0	0	12	8	23	16	35	24
19.07.04 - 08.10.04	0	0	0	0	0	0	5	4	4	4	9	8
16.12.04 - to date	4	4	4	2	13	8	4	1	66	22	91	37
Total	4	4	4	2	13	8	21	13	93	42	135	69

VIRUSES — AVIAN

Anatid Herpesvirus 1

Family Herpesviridae (Unassigned to a Genus): Anatid herpesvirus 1 is also known as duck enteritis virus or duck plague herpesvirus. Primary isolation of duck enteritis virus (DEV) is possible in DEF cells sourced from 19–20 day old embryonic Pekin, Muscovy, wood ducks, pintails, lesser scaup, black and red-head ducks, Pekin duck embryo fibroblast (ATCC no. CCL-141) cells, embryonated duck eggs (EDE) or ducklings. Primary DEF cell culture is more susceptible to DEV isolation than EDE, duckling or Pekin duck embryo fibroblast cell culture. Greatest sensitivity, highest viral titres and most obvious plaque formation are seen in DEF cells sourced from Muscovy and wood duck cells.

DEF cells sourced from Pekin, black and red-head ducks have intermediate sensitivity, and poor results are seen for DEF sourced from pintail and lesser scaup. Whilst DEF culture is reported to be the most sensitive isolation method there are reports of DEV field isolates that could not be isolated in DEF but were isolated by inoculation of ducklings and SN assay (Hanson and Willis 1976). The Pekin duck embryo fibroblast cell line has moderate sensitivity but plaque formation is indistinct (Barr et al. 1992; Kocan 1976; Lam and Lin 1986; OIE 2010; Shawky 2000; Shawky and Schat 2002; Shawky and Sandhu 1997).

Primary DEF cultures should be passaged 3 times prior to virus inoculation. Virus is adsorbed for 1 hour and the infected cultures are incubated for 3 days at 39.5–41.5 °C. CPE is evident as rounded, clumped cells that enlarge and become necrotic, formation of syncytia, intranuclear inclusions and granulation of the cytoplasm 48–96 hours after infection. Plaque formation is evident after 3 days for infected cell monolayers with agar overlays. Three passages are necessary to ensure detection of low levels of virus. Variability in growth characteristics is seen for different virus isolates and influences the efficacy of isolation, as well as the tendency for low levels of virus to establish persistent latent infection. Specific testing is recommended because of the difficulty of primary isolation of virus in cell culture.

Specific assays for DEV are FA, ISH, EM, SN, AC-ELISA, PCR, and real- time PCR.

A FA has been developed to confirm CPE in DEV-infected cultures using a fluorophore-conjugated mAb specific to DEV (Erickson et al. 1975; Proctor 1975). A SN assay has been developed that utilises either DEV-infected DEF monolayers or EDE. These assays have low sensitivity and are limited by the lack of an available standard positive anti-DEV serum.

A PCR has been developed for detection of DEV targeting the pol gene (Plummer et al. 1998). The PCR is combined with RFLP to confirm diagnosis. The PCR restriction fragment length polymorphism (PCR-RFLP) assay has a history of having been applied successfully to the diagnosis of DEV across wide geographic regions (Hansen et al. 1999; Hansen et al. 2000; Plummer et al. 1998; Pritchard et al. 1999). The PCR is reported to be highly specific for DEV and did not react with herpesviruses of other species. The PCR is reported to have a detection limit of 1 fg of genomic DNA and to be 20 times more sensitive than culture isolation alone (Hansen et al. 1999; Plummer et al. 1998).

The PCR has been adapted to a real-time Taqman PCR targeting the pol gene of DEV (Plummer et al. 1998; Qi et al. 2008a; Qi et al. 2008b; Yang et al. 2005). The Taqman assay has greater sensitivity and specificity than the PCR alone and the detection limit for the assay is 23 genomic copies. Molecular assays have the advantage of detection of latent inapparent infections.

The generalised culture methods of 9 CFR 113.52, 113.53 and 113.55 for extraneous agent testing will not be sufficient for primary isolation of DEV. The 9 CFR guidelines do not include specific testing for DEV.

The European Pharmacopoeia 2.6.24 Avian viral vaccines: tests for extraneous agents in seed lots do not provide guidelines for testing for antibodies in ducklings, but does specify SN assay for DEV. This method has been used for detection of clinical cases in numerous studies. The virus rapidly causes significant clinical disease within 3 days and seroconversion detectable by SN assay; however, the technique is problematic due to the failure to isolate all strains of DEV. The efficacy of this method has not been established for the detection of low levels of contaminating virus in biological products. A DEV- specific antiserum standard for the SN test and SPF ducklings can be difficult to obtain.

The generalised culture methods of 9 CFR 113.52, 113.53 and 113.55 are not acceptable.

Primary isolation of DEV in DEF sourced from Muscovy or wood duck is recommended. Primary DEF cultures should be passaged 3 times prior to virus inoculation. Virus is adsorbed for 1 hour, the infected cultures are incubated for 3 days at 39.5–41.5 °C, and 3 passages are required.

Specific testing is required for DEV by real-time Taqman PCR targeting the pol gene of DEV.

The method described by European Pharmacopoeia 2.6.24 is unreliable due to the failure to isolate all strains of DEV.

Avian Adenoviruses

Family Adenoviridae, genus Aviadenovirus and Atadenovirus: Avian isolates of adenoviruses comprise 2 genera: the genus Aviadenovirus encompasses serotypes 1, 2, 3, 4, 5, 6, 7, 8a, 8b, 9, 10 and 11, and the genus Atadenovirus encompasses the group III avian adenovirus, duck adenovirus A (egg drop syndrome (EDS) virus). Two parallel and different systems of nomenclature are in use by Europe and the United States to classify the serotypes of avian adenoviruses, complicating the correlation of serotype specific data.

A single system of nomenclature was adopted by the International Committee on Taxonomy of Viruses (ICTV) in 2006 and strain classification under this system has been cross referenced to the European and the United States nomenclature by (Büchen-Osmond 2006; Steer et al. 2009). Primary isolation of all serotypes of avian adenoviruses (AAdV) is possible in chicken embryo liver (CELi), CEF, CKC and chicken hepatoma (CH-SAH) cells. CH- SAH has been shown to be more sensitive than the conventional culture systems of CELi or CKC cells, and viral titres obtained are 2 logs higher than in other culture systems.

Susceptibility of CELi and chicken embryo kidney (CEK) cells is inconsistent between preparations and some isolates of AAdV have failed to grow in these cells. CEF is poorly susceptible to AAdV. Primary isolation of all viruses from mixed infections with more than 1 AAdV serotype have been reported to be successful from inoculation of ECE that were not able to be isolated from CH-SAH cell cultures (Ojkic et al. 2008). AAdV can form latent infections in culture and culture adaptation occurs. Primary isolation of AAdV may not be associated with gross evidence of CPE or pathology, therefore specific testing is required.

Specific testing is required for AAdV as some isolates establish inapparent infections in primary cultures. Specific testing is possible by agar gel precipitation (AGP), IFA, EIA, ELISA, RT-PCR or real-time RT-PCR.

When comparing serological methods the greatest sensitivity is achieved with the ELISA that targets the group specific antigen (GSA). The GSA is conserved within all 12 serotypes of AAdV group I (AAdV-I). ELISA for AAdV- I GSA has the advantages of high sensitivity (can detect 102 TCID50 virus) and broad-spectrum reactivity (Calnek et al. 1982; Saifuddin and Wilks 1990). The ELISA has significantly higher sensitivity than the AGP assay for detection of AAdV. Monreal and Dorn (1981) found in a parallel study that the ELISA was able to detect 47/55 samples as positive whereas the AGP could only detect 23/55 positives. Hess M (2000)reports ELISA detection of all 32 positive test samples of AAdV whereas AGP detected only 14 samples. Dawson et al (1982) report a significantly greater sensitivity for ELISA detection of AAdV than for EIA detection.

PCR has been developed for the detection of AAdV-I and AAdV group II (AAdV-II) based on the pol gene (Hanson et al. 2006; Jiang et al. 1999; Kumar et al. 2003; Moscoso et al. 2007; Pantin-Jackwood et al. 2007; Pantin-Jackwood et al. 2008; Persia et al. 2002; Toro et al. 1999; Wang et al. 2008; Xie and Khan 2000). The PCR is highly sensitive and specific, and has a threshold for detection of 1-10 fg of DNA.

The group III avian adenovirus, duck adenovirus A (EDS) is serologically unrelated to AAdV-I and AAdV-II and therefore specific testing for these viruses will not detect EDS. Specific testing for EDS is possible by HI, VN, HA, AC-ELISA or PCR. An AC-ELISA has been developed using F8 mAb specific to the hexon protein to capture EDS virus and polyclonal serum for detection (Dhinakar Raj et al. 2003). The sensitivity of the AC-ELISA for culture isolated EDS was 98 per cent and specificity was 96 per cent. A PCR assay targeting the J fragment of the EDS genome was shown to have equivalent sensitivity and specificity to the AC-ELISA, and both tests had 15 fold greater detection sensitivity when compared to HA test for 5 logs of virus (Dhinakar Raj et al. 2003).

The generalised culture methods of 9 CFR 113.52, 113.53 and 113.55 for extraneous agent testing will not be sufficient for primary isolation of AAdV- I. The 9 CFR guidelines do not include specific testing for AAdV.

The European Pharmacopoeia 2.6.24 refers to 3 methods for AAdV detection: primary isolation by inoculation of embryonic chickens 9-11 days old by the chorioallantoic, allantoic and yolk sac routes and examination after 7–12 days; inoculation of CKC and examination for CPE after culturing for 21 days and passaging at 4–7 day intervals; and inoculation of 2 week old chickens twice, at 2 week intervals and collection of serum. The serum is then tested for AAdV-I antibodies using the SN, EIA or AGP tests, and tested for egg drop syndrome virus using either haemagglutination inhibition (HI) or EIA. The sensitivity of these methods is significantly lower than culture isolation and specific testing by ELISA or PCR for AAdV-I.

The generalised culture methods of 9 CFR 113.52, 113.53 and 113.55 are not acceptable.

Primary isolation of AAdV-I in CH-SAH is recommended. Specific testing is required for AAdV-I by either ELISA or PCR. Specific testing is required for EDS by either AC-ELISA or PCR.

The methods described by European Pharmacopoeia 2.6.24 are not acceptable.

Avian Encephalomyelitis Virus

Family Picornaviridae, Genus Hepatovirus: Primary isolation of avian encephalomyelitis virus (AEV) is possible in CEF, baby grivet monkey kidney cells subclone (BGM-70), embryonic neuroglial cells, or by intracranial or allantoic inoculation of ECE. Growth is slow in allantoic fluid and better for intracranial inoculation of ECE. AEV will grow to only very low titres in CEF, and without evidence of CPE.

AEV can be grown in embryonic neuroglial cell cultures without evidence of CPE, but viral detection is possible using FA. AEV can also be propagated in the cell line BGM-70, but growth requires multiple passages before culture adaptation occurs. AEV that has been culture-adapted by initial passages in ECE has been shown to grow to relatively high titres in embryonic neuroglial cell lines. Isolation of AEV in chickens 2 weeks old followed by serological detection is of low sensitivity.

In general primary isolation combined with serological assays has poor specificity due to non-specific reactions and cross-reactions. Therefore specific testing is recommended. Specific testing for AEV is possible by AGP, EIA, AC-ELISA or RT-PCR.

The AGP test has the advantage of rapid detection of AEV antigen at 4 days after infection, but has very low sensitivity, and its specificity can be reduced by antigenic variability amongst AEV isolates. The sensitivity of the AC-ELISA test is better than that of the AGP, but is still too low for recommendation.

RT-PCR for AEV VP2 gene is highly sensitive and specific and can detect as little as 10 pg of viral RNA.

The generalised culture methods of 9 CFR 113.52, 113.53 and 113.55 for extraneous agent testing will not be sufficient for primary isolation of AEV. The 9 CFR guidelines do not include specific testing for AEV.

The European Pharmacopoeia 2.6.24 refers to general methods for detection of extraneous agents and specific methods for detection of AEV. The general methods are gross pathology and histopathology following inoculation of test material into the allantoic cavity, CAM and yolk sac of embryonated eggs, and by CPE detection in CKC monolayers. Specific isolation of AEV is by inoculation of chickens 2 weeks old and testing of serum for AEV by AGP or EIA. The sensitivity of both the general and specific methods is very low and they are not acceptable.

Avian Influenza Virus

Family Orthomyxoviridae, Genus Influenzavirus A: Primary isolation of avian influenza virus (AIV) is by allantoic inoculation of 9–11 day old embryonated SPF fowl eggs. The recommendation is for incubation of inoculated eggs for 4–7 days between passages. Allantoic fluid is harvested and tested for AIV. Allantoic fluid testing negative is passaged into fresh eggs at least 3 more times.

Specific testing is required to detect AIV in the allantoic fluid and HA and RT-PCR is recommended. Samples from the final passage together with an earlier passage should be tested.

The generalised culture method described in 9 CFR 113.37: Detection of pathogens by the chicken embryo inoculation test will not provide optimal growth conditions for AIV and will not be sufficient for isolation. The protocol 9 CFR 113.37 has a single passage in embryonated eggs, which is insufficient for isolation of low titre viruses. The 9 CFR guidelines do not include specific testing for AIV. The European Pharmacopoeia 2.6.24 specifies isolation of AIV by inoculation of chickens 2 weeks old and testing of serum for AIV by AGP or EIA. The European Pharmacopoeia 2.6.24 also includes requirements for generic detection of extraneous agents by gross pathology and histopathology following inoculation of test material into the allantoic cavity, CAM and yolk sac of embryonated eggs, and by CPE detection in CKC monolayers. The sensitivity of both the generic and specific methods is very low and they are not acceptable.

Avian Leukosis Virus

Family Retroviridae Genus Alpharetrovirus: Avian leukosis virus (ALV) comprises 6 subgroups on the basis of antigenic typing of the surface glycoprotein p27; subgroups A, B, C, D and J are transmitted as infectious viral particles and are classified as exogenous ALVs; subgroup

E is non-pathogenic, it is integrated into the genome of a high proportion of chickens and is classified as endogenous ALV. Subgroups A and B are highly prevalent, pathogenic exogenous viruses and are aetiological agents for clinical disease and oncogenesis. Subgroups C and D are rare exogenous viruses and subgroup J is a highly prevalent, severely pathogenic exogenous virus with a high transmission rate. Both endogenous and exogenous ALV can be transmitted vertically in biological materials originating from chickens.

ALV can be isolated by culture in CEF. CEF should be harvested from 9–11 day old embryos that are genetically susceptible to ALV subgroups A, B and J. CEF from C/E strain chickens are resistant to infection with endogenous ALV and support the growth of exogenous ALV. Super-infection of CEF with virus of a particular subgroup interferes with isolation of virus of that subgroup and CEF infected with ALV are not suitable for ALV culture isolation.

ALV is thermolabile and samples are required to be stored at –70 °C prior to inoculation into culture. Confluent monolayers of CEF of a susceptible phenotype should be inoculated with virus and adsorption incubation for 1 hour is required, followed by incubation for at least 21 days at 35–37 °C. Efficient propagation of ALV is highly dependent on optimal cell culture conditions, results can be unreliable and isolation requires several subcultures over at least 21 days.

In one report an unusual isolate of ALV subgroup A was obtained as a contaminant from commercial vaccines by culture isolation in CEF (Silva et al. 2007). The isolate was unusual in that virus growth was very, very slow in CEF and this was proposed to be due to the virus having an LTR sequence homologous with subgroup E viruses rather than subgroup A viruses. This report illustrates the potential difficulty of using the growth properties of exogenous viruses and detection methods developed for isolation of field strains for detecting vaccine contaminants which are atypical ALV isolates.

Specific testing for ALV is required because of the unreliability of culture isolation and because of the lack of discernable CPE for ALV-infected CEF. Most strains of ALV produce no visible morphological changes in cell culture assays (except after prolonged passage (Calnek 1968). Propagation of ALV is unreliable due to culture variables, CEF phenotypic resistance can inhibit virus growth, and super-infection of CEF with virus of the same subgroup can interfere with virus isolation. Specific testing for ALV is possible by methods that detect the GAG, POL or ENV viral proteins, or detect proviral DNA or viral RNA, or by enzyme bioassays.

Available assays based on detection of group specific viral protein are the Complement Fixation Assay for Avian Leukosis (COFAL (Sarma et al. 1964), ELISA (Crittenden et al. 1987; Fadly and Witter 1998; Smith et al.

1979), phenotypic mixing assay (PMA (Okazaki et al. 1979), Resistance-Inducing Factor (RIF) assay (Rubin 1960), Non-producer cell activation (NPA) (Rispens et al. 1970), direct and indirect FA and flow cytometry assays, and RIA (Estola et al. 1974; Sandelin et al. 1974). A limitation of assays based on detection of viral protein is that in general they do not distinguish between endogenous and exogenous ALV, because group-specific antigens can be produced by both types of virus. This limitation can be overcome in part by specialised culture techniques involving the use of combinations of CEF with phenotypes that are both sensitive and resistant to the different subgroups of ALV.

The COFAL and ELISA are the most commonly used assays. The COFAL test uses hamster serum (Sarma et al. 1964). Mammalian antiserum used in ELISA assays will detect all exogenous and endogenous strains of ALV whereas avian antiserum will be subgroup specific (Hunt et al. 2000; Hunt et al. 1999; Kelloff and Vogt 1966; Payne et al. 1966). Studies comparing the COFAL and ELISA assays have found that the sensitivity of the ELISA assay is greater than that of the COFAL assay. This is further supported by the finding that contamination of commercial vaccines with ALV has been detected by ELISA assay for samples that were found to be negative by COFAL assay.

The basis of the RIF assay is interference by virus of the same subgroup to result in at least a 10 times reduction in foci of the indicator infection with stock Rous sarcoma virus (RSV) (Rovigatti and Astrin 1983; Vogt and Ishizaki 1966). The usefulness of the RIF assay is limited to ALV isolates that are not rapidly cytopathic. The appearance of viral foci in the RIF test is very dependent on optimal cell culture conditions and results can be unreliable.

Non-producer cells are produced from CEF transformed with env-defective RSV (BH-RSV), then superinfection with leukosis helper virus results in detectable virus production. A variation of the test is infection of CEF cells with genotype susceptible to infection with endogenous and exogenous avian leukosis virus (C/O), with subgroup E RSV then superinfection with exogenous virus to produce detectable virus. The NPA test can also be performed using a Japanese quail cell line transformed by RSV that is high titre and ENV defective (R(-)Q) for assay of endogenous and exogenous ALV (Crittenden et al. 1979). The NPA test is a specialised technique and its use is limited by the availability of required phenotypes of CEF transformed with the defective BH-RSV. There are reports of false positive results when non-producer cells are coinfected with mixtures of complementing retroviruses (Zhang et al. 2008).

PCR and RT-PCR assays have been developed for ALV that mostly target sequence within the env locus or the LTR sequence. A subgroup-specific PCR assay has been developed for ALV subgroup A targeting the proviral DNA (Silva et al. 2007; van Woensel et al. 1992), and generic nested PCR and RT- PCR assays have been developed for detection of exogenous but not endogenous strains of ALV targeting the proviral conserved LTR and U5 sequences (Fadly and Witter 1998; García et al. 2003; Häuptli et al. 1997; Lupiani et al. 2000; Silva et al. 2000; Smith et al. 1998a; Smith et al. 1998b).

The nested RT-PCR and nested PCR assays were shown to be more sensitive than ELISA detection of cell culture isolated ALV (García et al. 2003). ALV subgroup A contamination of commercial poultry vaccines is reported to have been detected by nested RT-PCR assay in vaccine samples that were negative by culture isolation and COFAL assay, and were positive by ELISA assay only following thermal inactivation and dilution of samples to neutralise ELISA assay inhibitors (Zavala and Cheng 2006).

An assay for detection of surface ATPase activity has been developed for avian myeloblastosis virus (AMV); however, the assay is not useful for other types of avian retroviruses. All types and subgroups of ALV can be detected by the RT activity assay. The assay format has been adapted to a highly sensitive, PCR-based RT (PERT) assay. The PERT assay has been used to screen human vaccines that are produced in CEF or embryonated eggs in order to demonstrate freedom from avian retroviruses (Hussain et al. 2001; Tsang et al. 1999). As for human vaccines, the PERT assay could similarly be applied to the generic screening of veterinary vaccines for retrovirus contamination.

The 9 CFR 113.31 methods describe the detection of ALV by culture isolation in CEF followed by the COFAL testing for ALV subgroups A and B. The 9 CFR 113.31 protocol for isolation and specific testing for ALV will not be sufficient for detection of ALV.

The USDA Center for Veterinary Biologics Notice No. 03–13 was issued in 2003 to notify interested parties of contamination of a number of vaccines produced in North America and Europe with both exogenous and endogenous ALV. The vaccines were found to be contaminated with ALV by ELISA testing and were negative by the COFAL test, which is the current method outlined in 9 CFR 113.31. The USDA instigated proposed amendments to the testing requirements for ALV on January 31st 2007 (Docket No. APHIS–2007–0001). The proposed amendments to the 9 CFR 113.31 protocol are for ALV testing 'using a method that will detect extraneous replicating ALV and that is acceptable to APHIS'. The amendments do not specify testing requirements, simply that approval of the test is required by APHIS.

The European Pharmacopoeia 2.6.24 recommends culture isolation of ALV in CEF of a susceptible genotype for at least 9 days, followed by specific testing by either COFAL or ELISA assays. The protocol does not provide optimal culture conditions and the sensitivity of the COFAL test is unacceptably low.

Avian Nephritis Virus 1 And 2

Family Astroviridae, Genus Avastrovirus, Species Chicken Astrovirus: Primary isolation of avian nephritis virus (ANV) is possible in chicken hepatocellular carcinoma (LMH) and CKC cells or by inoculation of 1 day old chickens. Cell culture should be performed in serum-free medium. ANV is detected by plaque titration using agar overlays. The threshold dose detectable by experimental infection of chickens is 5 logs of virus, and therefore this method is not sufficiently sensitive for detection of the low levels of viral contaminants expected to be present in biologicals (Imada and Kawamura 1997; Mandoki 2006).

Irregular plaques are visible in CKC monolayers from 4 days after infection. CPE is evident as granular eosinophilic inclusions in the cytoplasm and virus can be detected by EM (Baxendale and Mebatsion 2004; Frazier 1990; Mandoki 2006; Takase et al. 1994).

The route of inoculation of ECE is a significant variable in the detection sensitivity; the order of sensitivity being inoculation by yolk sac, CAM, and lastly the allantoic route. The breed of chicken from which the CKC or ECE culture systems are derived also significantly affects the detection sensitivity (Baxendale and Mebatsion 2004; Frazier 1990).

ANV isolates vary in the CPE observed in culture systems. Non-cytopathic isolates of ANV have been described, and persistent culture infections are reported, characterised by low viral titres and absence of CPE. Specific testing is required to detect persistent or non-cytopathic ANV infections. Specific testing for ANV is possible by VN, AC-ELISA, FA, AGID and RT-PCR.

An FA has been developed for detection of ANV infected CKC monolayers on coverslips using virus specific mAbs (Baxendale and Mebatsion 2004; Imada et al. 1981; Imada et al. 1982; Mockett et al. 1993; Shirai et al. 1990; Takase 1989). A study systematically comparing serological detection of ANV reports the order of sensitivity of assays to be VN>ELISA>FA>AGID (Baxendale and Mebatsion 2004; Mockett et al. 1993). A RT-PCR assay targeting the gp1 gene has been developed for detection of ANV. The RT-PCR assay has a detection threshold of 10 copies of genome. Validation of the RT-PCR assay is reported for surveillance of chicken carcass samples, but the assay has not been sufficiently validated for diagnostic purposes (Baxendale and Mebatsion 2004; Mándoki et al. 2006; Pantin-Jackwood et al. 2008). The sequence hypervariability in the gp1 region is problematic for the design of molecular diagnostic assays that can detect all isolates (Mándoki et al. 2006). A multiplex RT-PCR assay has been developed for detection of ANV that can differentiate ANV from other astroviruses of chicken and turkey origin.

The generalised culture methods of 9 CFR 113.52, 113.53 and 113.55 for extraneous agent testing will not be sufficient for primary isolation of ANV. The 9 CFR guidelines do not include specific testing for ANV.

The European Pharmacopoeia 2.6.24 refers to general methods for detection of extraneous agents and specific methods for detection of ANV. The general methods are gross pathology and histopathology following inoculation of test material into the allantoic cavity, CAM and yolk sac of embryonated eggs, and by CPE detection in CKC monolayers. Specific isolation of ANV is by inoculation of chickens 2 week old and testing of serum for ANV by FA. Chickens are significantly more susceptible at 1 day old than 2 weeks old, and the sensitivity of this assay is inadequate for innocuity testing (Imada and Kawamura 1997; Mandoki 2006). The sensitivity of both the general and specific methods is very low and they are not acceptable.

AVIAN ORTHOREOVIRUS

Family Reoviridae, Genus Orthoreovirus

Avian orthoreovirus is more commonly known as avian reovirus. Primary isolation of avian reovirus is possible in CELi and CEF. Avian reovirus grows readily in CEF and forms identifiable plaques. The size and extent of plaques correlates with the virulence of the virus, with attenuated and low-pathogenic strains having reduced plaque formation in CEF. For these strains detection by inoculation of CEF is not sufficiently sensitive and specific testing is required.

Specific testing is possible by EM, IEM, FA, ELISA, RT-PCR and real- time RT-PCR. EM, FA and ELISA assays have low sensitivity and specificity.

A number of PCR assays have been developed for reovirus targeting different segments. A PCR assay has been developed for avian reoviruses targeting the S2 and S4 segments (Bruhn et al. 2005). The detection limit of the assay was 0.8 TCID50, the sensitivity for field isolates was 80 per cent and 55 per cent for the S4 and S2 targets respectively, and specificity was reported as 100 per cent. The assay was validated for use in extraneous agent testing of veterinary therapeutics. A multiplex real-time SYBR green RT-PCR assay has been developed for avian reoviruses to simultaneously detect sequence from the S1 segment of chicken–origin reovirus and from the S3 segment of turkey– origin reovirus (Ke et al. 2006; Spackman et al. 2005). The detection sensitivity for the real-time RT-PCR is greater than that recorded for virus isolation and for ELISA or FA, and 3 logs greater than for the classical RT-PCR assay. The real-time RT-PCR assay has a detection threshold of 39 copies/ml of genome and is highly sensitive and 100 per cent specific. The assay is highly reproducible and had minimal inter- and intra-assay variation. Variant and vaccine strains of reovirus can be differentiated using the melt curve analysis.

A nested PCR assay has also been described for avian reoviruses based on the sC gene on the S1 segment (Liu et al. 1997; Liu et al. 1999). The detection sensitivity of the classical PCR assay was 10 TCID50 and increased by 3 logs in the nested format.

The generalised culture methods of 9 CFR 113.52, 113.53 and 113.55 for extraneous agent testing will not be sufficient for primary isolation of avian reovirus. The 9 CFR guidelines do not include specific testing for avian reovirus.

The European Pharmacopoeia 2.6.24 refers to general methods for detection of extraneous agents by gross pathology and histopathology following inoculation of test material into the allantoic cavity, CAM and yolk sac of embryonated eggs, and by CPE detection in CKC monolayers. The European Pharmacopoeia 2.6.24 does not refer to specific testing for avian reovirus. The sensitivity of the general methods is very low and they are not acceptable.

Chicken Anaemia Virus

Family Circoviridae, Genus Gyrovirus: Primary isolation of chicken anaemia virus (CAV) is possible in Marek's disease virus (MDV) transformed chicken T lymphoblastoid (MDCC-MSB1 and MDCC-CU147) cell lines. MDCC-CU147 are reported to have 10 times greater detection sensitivity when compared to 26 MDV-transformed cell lines and are the most sensitive cell lines for primary isolation (Calnek et al. 2000).

FA is the diagnostic standard for flock surveillance; however, molecular assays have greater sensitivity and specificity for low level detection (McNeilly et al. 1991; Toro et al. 1997).

PCR and nested PCR assays have been developed targeting the VP1 gene of CAV (Imai et al. 1998; Miller et al. 2003; Tham and Stanislawek 1992a; Tham and Stanislawek 1992b). The detection limit of the assay is reported to be 10-1.5TCID50 (Imai et al. 1998). The assay sensitivity was increased by 100 times for the nested PCR assay (Imai et al. 1998; Soiné et al. 1993). PCR combined with dot blot hybridization using a radioactive probe has a detection sensitivity of 1 fg DNA (Todd et al. 1992). PCR assay is highly sensitive and specific and has been validated in a number of studies. The generalised culture methods of 9 CFR 113.52, 113.53 and 113.55 for extraneous agent testing will not be sufficient for primary isolation of CAV. The 9 CFR guidelines do not include specific testing for CAV.

The European Pharmacopoeia 2.6.24 refers to primary isolation of chicken anaemia virus in MDCC-MSB1 cells for at least 24 days and 8 passages followed by FA. PCR assay has been reported to be considerably more sensitive and specific than FA for culture-isolated CAV (Todd et al. 1992).

Duck Viral Hepatitis Virus 1

Family Picornaviridae (Unassigned to a Genus): There are at least 3 aetiological agents responsible for duck hepatitis. Duck viral hepatitis virus 1 (DVHV-1), is the most significant aetiological agent and the only agent considered here.

Primary isolation of DVHV-1 is possible in duck embryo liver (DEL), duck embryo kidney (DEK), DEF, EDE, and ducklings. The virus has poor growth in cell culture and only grows to low titres. The latent period for virus growth is 24 hours and several passages are required to ensure detection. CPE is not obvious and specific detection is required. An adsorption incubation of 30 minutes is required for virus inoculation onto DEL monolayers. DEL is more susceptible to DVHV-1 growth than DEK or DEF cell cultures (Hwang 1965; Hwang 1966). Plaque formation is more readily identified for cell culture- adapted virus isolates, whereas more virulent field isolates may grow in DEL without evidence of CPE or plaque formation (Woolcock 1986). Virus growth can be identified by FA or RT-PCR methods in these non-cytopathic cultures. Culture-adapted isolates are also less sensitive to growth inhibition by serum components.

A multi-stage isolation process is most successful for DVHV-1 to ensure culture adaptation occurs. Isolation of DVHV-1 is by initial subcutaneous or intramuscular inoculation of 1–7 day old SPF ducklings. Characteristic clinical signs and death occur within 18–48 hours and virus is then re-isolated from liver homogenised in 20 per cent buffered saline with 5 per cent chloroform added. The second stage of the isolation process is allantoic inoculation of the harvested liver homogenate into 10–14 day old EDE and virus is re-isolated from the liver of embryos at 72 hours.

EDE are more susceptible to DVHV-1 than ECE, and ECE are not recommended for primary isolation of DVHV-1. Alternatively, the second stage isolation can also be performed in DEL cells which are highly susceptible to DVHV-I (Woolcock et al. 1982; Woolcock 1986). DVHV-I infection of DEL monolayers with agarose overlays produces 1mm diameter plaques at 24 hours. Serum or foetal calf serum at concentrations £ 0.1 per cent in the growth medium reduces DVHV-1 plaque formation and at concentrations e" 0.2 per cent inhibits virus growth completely. The non-specific growth inhibition by mammalian serum components on DVHV-1 is attributed to an effect of the albumen fraction on the virus itself, rather than on virus attachment to cell culture receptors and virus entry (Chalmers and Woolcock 1984; OIE 2010; Woolcock et al. 1982; Woolcock 1986). Specific testing for DVHV-1 is required due to the difficulty of primary isolation and the high frequency of non- cytopathic isolates in DEL culture.

Specific testing for DVHV-1 is possible by FA, SN, AGID, immunohistochemical assay (IHA), ELISA, RT-PCR, and real-time RT-PCR.

The SN test is performed either in ovo or as a plaque reduction assay in vitro using hyperimmune duck serum (Woolcock 1986). Caution should be used in the interpretation of the SN assay to control for the common occurrence of non-specific growth inhibition of DVHV-1 by serum components (Chalmers and Woolcock 1984). The SN test suffers from non-specific reactions and false positives and variability for repetitions of the assay.

A study comparing the performance of the ELISA, SN and AGID tests for detection of DVHV-1 found equivalent specificity for all 3 tests; however, the sensitivities of the assays were 68.8 per cent, 68.8 per cent and 18.8 per cent respectively (Zhao et al. 1991).

A one-step RT-PCR assay has been developed that detects the pol (3D) gene of DVHV-1 with 100 per cent specificity and a detection threshold of either 10 median embryo lethal doses (ELD50)/ml, 100 pg RNA or 103 viral genomic copies (Kim et al. 2008a; Kim et al. 2007a)). A SYBR green real-time RT-PCR assay has been developed for DVHV-1 combined with a melting curve analysis to demonstrate specificity, with a reported 100 per cent sensitivity and 100 per cent specificity (Wang et al. 2002). The RT-PCR and real-time SYBR green RT-PCR assays have not been adequately validated for diagnostic purposes.

The generalised culture methods of 9 CFR 113.52, 113.53 and 113.55 for extraneous agent testing will not be sufficient for primary isolation of DVHV-1. The 9 CFR guidelines do not include specific testing for DVHV-1.

The European Pharmacopoeia 2.6.24 requires inoculation of 1 day old ducklings followed by SN assay for DVHV-1. The SN test has low specificity, poor repeatability and interpretation of output from the SN assay is problematic.

Fowlpox Virus

Family Poxviridae, Genus Avipoxvirus: Primary isolation of fowlpox virus is possible in CEF, CEK, chicken embryo dermis and quail fibrosarcoma (QT-35) cells, or ECE. CPE is readily visible as large intracytoplasmic inclusion bodies (Bollinger bodies) that contain smaller elementary bodies (Borrel bodies) in haematoxylin and eosin (H&E) stained preparations. EM can be used to confirm the presence of pox viruses with characteristic morphology. Some attenuated strains of fowlpox virus do not form obvious plaques in cell culture. Fowlpox virus requires cell culture adaptation to grow in primary chicken cell lines such as CEF, CEK, QT-35 or dermal cells. Fowlpox virus isolates can form latent infections and atypical fowlpox virus is difficult to diagnose.

Fowlpox virus can be isolated by inoculation onto the CAM of 9–12 day old ECE, incubation for 5–7 days, and then examination for small focal white pock lesions (OIE 2010). Specific testing is required to confirm virus detection. Specific testing is by FA, EM, ELISA, AGID, HI, immunoblot, DNA hybridization, or PCR.

FA and EM assays are used to confirm CPE or pock formation in infected cultures. The AC-ELISA is 400–800 times more sensitive than the AGID test for serological detection in inoculated embryos (Zhang et al. 2005).

A PCR assay has been developed for fowlpox virus targeting the 4b core protein (Lee and Lee 1997). The detection threshold for the PCR assay was 10-1 TCID50 or 150 genomic copies. A nested PCR has been developed that uses as external primers those used by Lee and Lee (1997) and an internal pair of primers (Fallavena et al. 2002). The nested PCR format increased the detection sensitivity relative to the classical PCR assay and the detection threshold was 0.28 EID50. Specificity of the nested PCR was established using a range of other pox viruses. The nested PCR assay was sufficiently sensitive to detect low titre infections such as chronic or latent fowlpox virus infections that were not detectable by the classical PCR assay. The generalised culture methods of 9 CFR 113.52, 113.53 and 113.55 for extraneous agent testing will not be sufficient for primary isolation of fowlpox virus. The 9 CFR guidelines do not include specific testing for fowlpox virus.

The European Pharmacopoeia does not have specific testing requirements for fowlpox virus beyond generalized extraneous agent testing. The European Pharmacopoeia 2.6.24 refers to general methods for detection of extraneous agents by gross pathology and histopathology following inoculation of test material into the allantoic cavity, CAM and yolk sac of embryonated eggs, and by CPE detection in CKC monolayers. The sensitivity of the general methods is very low and they are not acceptable.

Infectious Bronchitis Virus

Family Coronaviridae, Genus Coronavirus : Primary isolation of infectious bronchitis virus (IBV) is possible in 9–11 days and used to re-inoculate ECE. Three serial passages in embryos are required. Growth of IBV in embryos is evident by teratogenic pathology and specific testing is required to confirm IBV infection. FA using a group-specific mAb is used to identify virus infection of the CAM. IBV can grow in TOC but this method is not recommended for primary isolation. IBV requires culture adaptation by passage in eggs before isolates will grow in tissue culture with identifiable CPE. TOC are prepared as suspensions of tissue from 20 day old ECE and can be used for infection of culture-adapted IBV(OIE 2010).

Specific assays for IBV are real-time RT-PCR, RT-PCR combined with RFLP, immunoblot, EIA, AGID, FA, HI, VN, or ELISA.

The AGID test lacks sensitivity and HI and ELISA have poor reproducibility and low sensitivity. Specific testing of the allantoic fluid from IBV infected ECE is possible by RT-PCR, detection by a DNA probe in a dot blot hybridization assay, FA, ELISA or ISH. MAbs used for detection of IBV in FA, ELISA, VN or ISH assays are limited in application by the continued emergence of new antigenic types of IBV that are not reactive (Karaca et al. 1992). ELISA is the most sensitive serological assay available for IBV (Hawkes et al. 1983; Karaca et al. 1992; Mockett and Darbyshire 1981).

A RT-PCR assay has been developed targeting the S1 subunit of the spike gene of IBV (Jackwood et al. 1997). The spike gene encodes a hypervariable region of the genome that correlates with the intra-species variation in neutralising antigenic epitopes. The RT-PCR assay is combined with RFLP for typing of virus isolates (Abreu et al. 2006; Jackwood et al. 2005; Jackwood et al. 2007). The assay specificity is enhanced by the inclusion of an internal control RNA, and the assay is sufficiently sensitive to detect IBV from field samples without the necessity for primary isolation in ECE. The assay has been adapted to a real-time SYBR green RT-PCR assay; however, this assay has not been sufficiently validated and the sensitivity or specificity of the assay has not been established for diagnostic purposes (Pantin-Jackwood et al. 2005). A 1 step real-time fluorogenic RT-PCR assay has been developed targeting ORF 1b, for generic detection of coronaviruses, including IBV (Escutenaire et al. 2007). The generic coronavirus real-time RT-PCR has a detection threshold of 10 genomic copies, is reported to detect 32 different species of coronavirus, and is highly specific to coronaviruses.

The generalised culture methods of 9 CFR 113.52, 113.53 and 113.55 for extraneous agent testing will not be sufficient for primary isolation of IBV. The 9 CFR guidelines do not include specific testing for IBV.

The European Pharmacopoeia 2.6.24 refers to inoculation of 2 week old chickens followed by EIA or HI assay for IBV. This method is not recommended due to the high frequency of failures for isolation of IBV in 2 week old chickens and the low sensitivity of detection of seroconversion by EIA and HI (de Wit 2000). Newly emergent antigenic variants of IBV occur at high frequency and will not be detected by the EIA method. The European Pharmacopoeia 2.6.24 also refers to general methods for detection of extraneous agents by gross pathology and histopathology following inoculation of test material into the allantoic cavity, CAM and yolk sac of embryonated eggs, and by CPE detection in CKC monolayers. The sensitivity of both the general and specific methods is very low and they are not acceptable.

Infectious Bursal Disease Virus

Family Birnaviridae, Genus Avibirnavirus: There are 2 serotypes of infectious bursal disease virus (IBDV): serotype 1 is pathogenic for poultry and is the serotype targeted by diagnostic assays, whereas serotype 2 is not pathogenic for poultry.

Primary isolation of IBDV is possible in QT-35, Vero, BGM-70, chicken B- lymphoblastoid cell lines transformed by Rous-associated virus 2 (LSCC-RP9 and LSCC-RP12), chicken macrophage (MQ-NCSU), B-lymphoblastoid cells, ECE, or CEF cultures. ECE, CEF, BGM-70, Vero and QT-35 cell lines are most frequently used for IBDV isolation. IBDV infected cultures should be incubated for 3 days and passaged at least 3 times to ensure detection. CPE is apparent at 48--72 hours as cellular aggregation, rounding, granulation and necrosis with plaque formation in monolayers of cells (OIE 2010).

Attempts at primary isolation of IBDV in chickens at 2 and 3 weeks of age showed variable success and resulted in a high frequency of false negatives (Abdel-Alim and Saif 2001b). IBDV inoculation of 1 day old chickens has lower detection sensitivity than inoculation of ECE (Abdel-Alim and Saif 2001b).

IBDV serotype 1 strains are classified as classical (cIBDV), variant (vIBDV) or very virulent (vvIBDV). Some isolates of vvIBDV require passaging in ECE and cannot be adapted to growth in QT-35, Vero, BGM-70, LSCC-RP9, MQ- NCSU, LSCC-RP12, or B-lymphoblastoid cells (Abdel-Alim and Saif 2001a; Hussain and Rasool 2005).

IBDV undergoes culture-adaptation and attenuation with serial passages in cell culture. Culture-adaptation has been associated with changes in 3 residues of the VP2 structural protein.

Culture-adapted isolates are difficult to detect as they have reduced pathogenicity indices in ECE or in chickens, and reduced CPE in cell culture. Several studies report that IBDV infection could not be detected in chickens by IEM, IF, AC-ELISA or RT-PCR following inoculation with a culture adapted virus (Abdel-Alim and Saif 2001b). Specific testing for IBDV is therefore required because of the difficulties of primary isolation. Specific testing for IBDV is possible by AC-ELISA, IEM, AGP, VN, IP, FA, RT-PCR or real-time RT-PCR assays. day old ECE by allantoic inoculation. The allantoic fluid is cullected ater 3-7 with the full range of IBDV strains.

The ELISA is the most sensitive of the immunological techniques but has lower sensitivity than molecular assays. Cross reaction of serotype 2, non-pathogenic IBDV has been reported for the 5 commercially available ELISA kits, limiting their usefulness for IBDV serotype 1 detection (Hussain and Rasool 2005).

A number of RT-PCR and real-time RT-PCR assays have been developed with very high sensitivity and specificity. A RT-PCR assay targeting the VP4 gene of IBDV failed to differentiate between serotype 1 and 2 (Wu et al. 1992). A RT-PCR assay has been developed for IBDV detection targeting the VP2 structural gene sequence that is specific for serotype 1 (Lin et al. 1994). This assay was adapted to a slot-blot format and also adapted to a QC-PCR assay (Akin et al. 1993; Wu et al. 1997). The VP2 region amplified in the RT-PCR assay incorporates a hypervariable region used for identification of strain markers by RT-PCR-RE and RT-PCR-RFLP assays (Akin et al. 1993; Jackwood et al. 2003; Jackwood and Sommer 2002; Jackwood and Sommer 2005; Lin et al. 1994; Peters et al. 2005; Sapats and Ignjatovic 2002; Wu et al. 1997; Wu et al. 2007). It has not been possible to identify markers that consistently identify IBDV strains according to pathotypes. The RT-PCR assay has been further adapted to a SYBR green real-time RT-PCR assay targeting the VP2 gene (Li et al. 2007).

Another real-time Taqman RT-PCR assay has been developed utilising probes specific to the classical, variant and virulent groups of virus and targeting the VP4 gene sequence (Peters et al. 2005). The real-time Taqman RT-PCR assay targeting the VP4 gene had 100 per cent specificity for IBDV serotype 1 and a detection threshold of 300 genomic copies. A fluorescence resonance energy transfer (FRET) real-time RT-PCR assay targeting the VP2 gene has been developed that is used to differentiate between the subgroups of IBDV by melt curve analysis and this assay has been used for diagnostic surveillance (Jackwood et al. 2003).

The generalised culture methods of 9 CFR 113.52, 113.53 and 113.55 for extraneous agent testing will not be sufficient for primary isolation of IBDV. The 9 CFR guidelines do not include specific testing for IBDV.

The European Pharmacopoeia 2.6.24 refers to general methods for detection of extraneous agents and specific methods for detection of IBDV. The general methods are gross pathology and histopathology following inoculation of test material into the allantoic cavity, CAM and yolk sac of embryonated eggs, and by CPE detection in CKC monolayers. Specific isolation of IBDV is by inoculation of chickens 2 weeks old followed by AGP, EIA or VN assay for IBDV. Inoculation of 2 week old chickens has an unacceptably high failure rate and will not be sufficiently sensitive for isolation of culture- adapted strains (Abdel-Alim and Saif 2001b). The AGP, EIA and VN assays have lower sensitivity than the molecular assays described above. The sensitivity of both the general and specific methods is very low and they are not acceptable.

Infectious Laryngotracheitis Virus

Family Herpesviridae, Genus Iltovirus: The taxonomically correct name for Infectious laryngotracheitis virus is gallid herpesvirus 1. Primary isolation of infectious laryngotracheitis virus (ILTV) is possible in ECE, CELi, CEK or CKC cells. CELi cells are the most sensitive culture system for ILTV isolation. Infected cultures require 2 hours incubation to allow virus adsorption to cells, and cultures are then incubated for 7 days and examined daily for evidence of CPE. Three blind passages in culture are required for isolation. CPE is evident as the formation of syncytia and intranuclear inclusions. CPE can be confirmed by FA using hyperimmune, polyclonal chicken antiserum or mAbs specific to ILTV, to stain the intranuclear inclusions (Ide 1978). Isolation in ECE is by inoculation onto the dropped CAM of 10–12 day old ECE. The CAM is examined for pock formation at 7 days after inoculation (OIE 2010).

ILTV can establish persistent, latent, low–level, inapparent infections of infected cultures that are difficult to detect. Primary isolation of ILTV can be inhibited by overgrowth with bacteria or adenovirus (Williams et al. 1994). Specific testing is required because of the high frequency of false negative results for culture isolation of ILTV.

Specific testing is possible by FA, EM, AGID, ELISA, SN and nested PCR. FA using a polyclonal hyperimmune antiserum from convalescent chickens has good sensitivity for virulent strains but a high rate of false negatives for avirulent or attenuated strains of ILTV (Ide 1978). The FA has poor repeatability between laboratories and strains.

A PCR assay was developed for ILTV targeting the tk gene (Abbas et al. 1996). The specificity of the PCR assay was increased by combining it with a hybridization assay using a biotinylated DNA probe. The PCR assay demonstrated 100 per cent specificity when tested against the CELi culture and a range of avian pathogens. The specificity of the DNA probe hybridization assay was highly dependent on the stringency of the assay conditions. The detection limit for the PCR assay was 1 mg DNA.

A nested PCR assay has been developed for detection of ILTV targeting the unique short region of the genome (Humberd et al. 2002). The nested PCR assay is reported to have 100 per cent specificity when tested against a panel of avian pathogens, and a detection threshold of 50–500 fg/ml of DNA. The sensitivity of virus isolation was 33 per cent greater when compared to molecular detection by nested PCR, and the molecular assay could detect ILTV 1994). A number of PCR-RFLP assays have been developed for ILTV targeting the tk, gC, glycoprotein X (gX), and ICP4 genes, with the objective of differentiating between field and vaccine strains of ILTV (Chang et al. 1997; Graham et al. 2000; Han and Kim 2001a; Han and Kim 2001b). The ICP4 gene has the greatest polymorphism of the tested target genes and is therefore the most useful target for strain discrimination (Chang et al. 1997). The detection limit for the PCR assay targeting ICP4 was 30 pg DNA or 10 PFU, and the assay was found to be 100 per cent specific. The PCR-RFLP assay targeting the ICP4 gene has been successfully applied to diagnostic surveys of ILTV strains across wide geographic areas.

The PCR-RFLP assay has been adapted to a real-time SYBR green PCR- RFLP assay targeting the ICP4 gene and combined with a melt curve analysis (Creelan et al. 2006; Johnson et al. 1995). The assay is reported to have 100 per cent specificity for ILTV strains, and is combined with RFLP analysis to include strain discrimination. The detection threshold of the real-time SYBR green PCR assay is 140 genomic copies/µl and the assay had 100 per cent sensitivity for detection of field cases of ILTV.

The generalised culture methods of 9 CFR 113.52, 113.53 and 113.55 for extraneous agent testing will not be sufficient for primary isolation of ILTV. The 9 CFR guidelines do not include specific testing for ILTV.

The European Pharmacopoeia 2.6.24 refers to general methods for detection of extraneous agents and specific methods for detection of ILTV. The general methods are gross pathology and histopathology following inoculation of test material into the allantoic cavity, CAM and yolk sac of embryonated eggs, and by CPE detection in CKC monolayers. Specific isolation of ILTV is by inoculation of 2 week old chickens followed by SN, EIA or FA for ILTV. Inoculation of 2 week old chickens is less sensitive than isolation in ECE or CELi cells. Specific testing by SN, EIA or FA is not suitable due to the high rate of false negative results with these tests. The sensitivity of both the general and specific methods is very low and they are not acceptable.

Marek's Disease Virus 1 and 2

Family Herpesviridae, Genus Mardivirus: The taxonomically correct name for Marek's disease virus 1 and 2 is gallid herpesvirus 2 and 3 respectively. Primary isolation of MDV is possible on CKC, DEF and CEF. DEF cells are the most sensitive culture system for detection of MDV-1. The inoculum is adsorbed for 40 minutes prior to the addition of maintenance medium. Plaque formation occurs within 3 days of inoculation and can be confirmed by FA using mAbs specific to MDV-1 (Lee et al. 1983). Cultures are maintained for 7 days with medium changed every 2 repeatability due to latency of virus (OIE 2010). MDV is highly cell-associated and cannot be purified in a cell–free medium. Specific testing is required due to the difficulty of primary isolation.

Specific testing is possible by PCR, AGID, FA, VN and ELISA. Serological diagnosis of MDV is problematic as turkey herpesvirus (HVT) shares common antigens with MDV and HVT cross reacts in serological assays (Davidson et al. 1991; Davidson et al. 1995a).

A PCR assay has been developed for MDV-1 targeting the 132 bp tandem repeat located in the BamHI-H fragment of the genome (Becker et al. 1992; Becker et al. 1993; Davidson et al. 1995b; Davidson et al. 2002; Zhu et al. 1992). The size of the PCR product is dependent on the number of repeats present and correlates with the virulence of the isolate as either an oncogenic or attenuated strain. The PCR assay targeting the 132 bp tandem repeat region is reported to have 100 per cent specificity for MDV-1 and was more sensitive than virus isolation for detection of MDV-1 in commercial flocks (Davidson et al. 1995b).

A second target for PCR assays for MDV detection has been the ICP4 gene, and this assay has been adapted to a quantitative competitive PCR (QC- PCR) using fluorescent primers (Anderson et al. 1992; Bumstead et al. 1997; Burgess and Davison 1999). The detection limit for the QC-PCR is reported to be 40 copies of DNA but the assay range was too narrow to be useful. The QC- PCR assay had reasonable repeatability with 15 per cent variance between replicate results, and was 100 per cent specific to MDV-1 (Bumstead et al. 1997).

A QC-PCR assay was developed targeting the gB gene of MDV and using a competitor DNA fragment (Reddy et al. 2000). The assay detection limit was 5 fg DNA and it was 100 per cent specific to MDV. Because MDV is highly cell-associated it is difficult to establish the detection limit of the assay relative to a bioassay for MDV.

The generalised culture methods of 9 CFR 113.52, 113.53 and 113.55 for extraneous agent testing will not be sufficient for primary isolation of MDV. The 9 CFR guidelines do not include specific testing for MDV.

The European Pharmacopoeia 2.6.24 refers to general methods for detection of extraneous agents and specific methods for detection of MDV. The general methods are gross pathology and histopathology following inoculation of test material into the allantoic cavity, CAM and yolk sac of embryonated eggs, and by CPE detection in CKC monolayers. Specific isolation of MDV is by inoculation of 2 week old chickens and testing of serum by AGP. The sensitivity of both the general and specific methods is very low and they are not acceptable. The European Pharmacopoeia 2.6.25 Avian live virus vaccines: tests for extraneous agents in batches of finished product refers to primary isolation of MDV in CEF cultivated for 21 days in which there are at least 3 passages. The cultures are tested by FA using a MDV-specific mAb. Isolation in CEF is less sensitive than in DEF or CKC.

Newcastle Disease Virus

Family Paramyxoviridae, Genus Avulavirus: Primary isolation of Newcastle disease virus (NDV) is by allantoic inoculation of 9–11 day old embryonated SPF fowl eggs. The recommendation is for incubation of inoculated eggs for 4–7 days between passages. Allantoic fluid is harvested and tested for NDV. Allantoic fluid testing negative is passaged into fresh eggs at least 3 more times.

Specific testing is required to detect NDV in the allantoic fluid. Specific testing for NDV is recommended by HA and RT-PCR assays on samples from the final passage together with an earlier passage.

The generalised culture method described in 9 CFR 113.37: Detection of pathogens by the chicken embryo inoculation test will not provide optimal growth conditions for NDV and will not be sufficient for isolation of NDV. The protocol 9 CFR 113.37 has an incubation period of 7 days for the inoculated eggs, which is insufficient for isolation of low titre viruses. The 9 CFR guidelines do not include specific testing for NDV detection. The European Pharmacopoeia 2.6.24 refers to general methods for detection of extraneous agents and specific methods for detection of NDV. The general methods are gross pathology and histopathology following inoculation of test material into the allantoic cavity, CAM and yolk sac of embryonated eggs, and by CPE detection in CKC monolayers. Specific isolation is inoculation of chickens 2 weeks old and testing of serum by HI and EIA. The sensitivity of both the general and specific methods is very low and they are not acceptable.

Reticuloendotheliosis Virus

Family Retroviridae, Genus Gammaretrovirus: Primary isolation of reticuloendotheliosis virus (REV) is possible in DEF, CEF and 1 day old SPF chickens. CPE can be detected in infected CEF 5 days after inoculation and is confirmed by FA using mAbs (Bagust and Dennet 1977). REV isolates may establish non-cytolytic infections that are difficult to detect, and therefore specific testing is required.

Specific testing is possible by FA, ELISA, complement fixation procedure for assay of avian REV (COFAR), PCR and real-time PCR.

Therefore PCR detection in conjunction with the FA and primary isolation is recommended.

A PCR assay has been developed targetting the LTR region of REV (Aly et. al. 1993). The PCR has been shown to be at least 10 times more sensitive than FA. FA and PCR were reported to be more sensitive than ELISA for detection of REV isolated in CEF, whereas ELISA was most sensitive for detection of REV isolated in chickens(Fadly and Witter 1997). A second PCR assay has been developed for REV targeting the env gene and is reported to have equivalent sensitivity to the assay targeting the LTR in direct comparisons (Davidson and Malkinson 1996). The detection limit for the PCR assay targeting the ENV gene was found to be 23.5 pg and when combined with a hybridization probe the limit of detection was 2.35 pg.

A real-time SYBR green PCR assay has also been developed for detection of REV targeting the regions encoding the ENV and the LTR (Tadese et al. 2008). Confirmation of assay specificity is achieved by melt curve analysis or sequencing. The real-time assay was reported to be 100 per cent specific for REV and the detection limit was 3–5 target copies. Adaption of this assay to either MGB or FRET probes did not increase the assay sensitivity but did allow strain discrimination for REV. The real-time SYBR green RT-PCR assay has greater sensitivity than FA assay.

Contamination of veterinary vaccines with REV has been a significant source of virus infection in vaccinated chickens and extraneous agent testing for REV is therefore an important consideration (Fadly and Witter 1997). REV contamination of fowl pox virus vaccines is due to integrated REV provirus in the fowl pox virus genome (Bagust and Dennet 1977; Bendheim 1973; Tadese et al. 2008). A real-time SYBR green PCR method has been developed for differentiation of the REV integrated into the fowl pox virus genome from non-fowl pox virus associated provirus targeting the integration site of fowl pox virus-REV (Tadese et al. 2008).

The generalised culture methods of 9 CFR 113.52, 113.53 and 113.55 for extraneous agent testing will not be sufficient for primary isolation of REV. The 9 CFR guidelines do not include specific testing for REV.

The European Pharmacopoeia 2.6.24 specifies primary isolation of REV in CEF cultivated for at least 10 days in which there were at least 3 passages. Virus is detected by FA staining of monolayers at the third passage. The method described by European Pharmacopoeia 2.6.24 will not detect non-cytolytic infections.

Turkey Rhinotracheitis Virus

Family Paramyxoviridae, Genus Metapneumovirus: The taxonomically correct name for turkey rhinotracheitis virus is avian metapneumovirus; however, it is also known as avian pneumovirus. The most sensitive method for the primary isolation of turkey rhinotracheitis virus (TRV) is a 2-stage isolation process in ECE and Vero cells. In the first stage, sample is inoculated into the yolk sac of 6 day old ECE. Allantoic fluid and yolk sac are harvested 8 days later, homogenised and used for 3 serial passages in ECE (Cook and Cavanagh 2002).

In the second stage, the egg fluid is harvested and homogenised and is then inoculated onto Vero, CELi or CEF. Vero cells are more sensitive than

CEF or CELi for the second stage of isolation. CPE in Vero cells is readily evident as pinpoint foci of cytolysis at 5 days after inoculation, cytoplasmic eosinophilic inclusions and polykaryocytes. Some isolates fail to grow in monolayer cultures or establish inapparent non-cytolytic infections. Specific testing is therefore required.

Alternatively primary isolation is possible in TOC. Four passages at 4 day intervals are required in TOC, because initially there is ciliostasis and inhibition of culture propagation. The inhibitory effect on TOC can give unreliable results and therefore the 2-stage isolation method in ECE and Vero cells is recommended as the method of choice (Cook and Cavanagh 2002).

Specific testing for TRV is possible by FA, EM, EIA, ELISA and RT-PCR. FA, EM, ELISA and EIA are reported to have low detection sensitivities and are not suitable for extraneous agent testing.

FA can be used to confirm TRV-induced CPE in infected monolayers. This technique has been applied widely to studies of TRV; however, there have been a number of formats for the assays used and there has not been a consistent study to establish the validity of the assay and its sensitivity and specificity for TRV diagnosis (Baxter-Jones et al. 1986; Cook 2000; Jones et al. 1986; Jones et al. 1987). The FAs developed have used turkey convalescent sera (Jones et al. 1988), hyperimmune serum raised in rabbits (Majó et al. 1995; O'Loan and Allan 1990) or mouse-anti-TRT mAbs (Catelli et al. 1998; Cook 2000).

There are a number of subtypes of TRV: A, B, C, D, E and F. A RT-PCR assay has been developed that is capable of detecting all subtypes of TRV, targeting the N gene, and combined with a G gene-based sub-typing RT-PCR assay (Bäyon-Auboyer et al. 1999). Other RT-PCRs have been developed that are subtype specific. In a comparison of RT-PCR targets, it is reported that only the assay targeting the N gene had 100 per cent sensitivity for isolates obtained from 4 different countries (Bäyon-Auboyer et al. 1999). The RT-PCR targeting the N gene detected 100 per cent of samples tested, whereas in direct comparison Vero cell culture isolation detected only 27 per cent and ELISA detection from experimental infections detected only 63 per cent of positives (Bäyon-Auboyer et al. 1999).

The generalised culture methods of 9 CFR 113.52, 113.53 and 113.55 for extraneous agent testing will not be sufficient for primary isolation of TRV. The 9 CFR guidelines do not include specific testing for TRV.

The European Pharmacopoeia 2.6.24 refers to primary isolation of TRV in chickens 2 weeks old followed by EIA on serum. The sensitivity of primary isolation in chickens 2 weeks old is low and this method is therefore not suitable for extraneous agent testing (Cook and Cavanagh 2002). The European Pharmacopoeia 2.6.25 part 5 refers to testing for TRV in CEF monolayers from 9 day old embryos followed by FA. CEF cells have lower sensitivity than Vero cells for TRV isolation.

BACTERIA — BRUCELLA SPP.

Brucella Abortus

Detection of Brucella spp. is based on the growth of characteristic 1–2 mm pearly white, round colonies on tellurite glycine agar (TGA) by 4 days. Uniform coccobacilli are found on bacterial smears, which are not acid-fast but resistant to decolourisation using Stamp's stain.

Low levels of Brucella spp. may not be detected on TGA due to overgrowth by other agents. Inhibition by components of the test material such as lipid droplets is a significant consideration for the testing of vaccine materials as adjuvants are mostly lipid-based formulations. It is recommended that isolation is performed in selective medium to reduce overgrowth and inoculation of enrichment medium to increase sensitivity of detection. The most widely used selective medium for isolation of Brucella abortus is Farrell's medium which is prepared by the addition of 6 antimicrobials (polymyxin B sulphate, bacitracin, natamycin, nalidixic acid, nystatin, and vancomycin) to the basal medium. The addition of 2–5 per cent equine or bovine serum is necessary for the growth of strains such as B. abortus biovar 2. Incubation of cultures should be at 37 °C and in 5–10 per cent CO2 for up to 6 weeks. Colony identification is by the following biochemical tests; urease, oxidase and catalase tests. A slide agglutination test is then conducted using anti-Brucella polyclonal serum. However, the slide agglutination test has poor specificity (OIE 2010; Roop, II et al. 1987).

Specific testing for B. abortus is recommended by either immune staining with a fluorochrome-conjugated mAb or by PCR. A colony blot ELISA that uses the mAb BRU 38 directed against the O side chain of lipopolysaccharide (LPS) is rapid, highly sensitive and has greatly improved specificity for detection of B. abortus.

Brucella genus-specific PCR assays directed against either the BCSP31 or 16S ribosomal RNA (rRNA) genes have been developed and standardised and are widely used. These PCR assays will not distinguish between the 6 species of the Brucella genus. Species specific and biovar specific B. abortus assays are mostly based on single nucleotide polymorphisms. The multi-locus AMOS PCR targeting the ery locus of Brucella spp. (AMOS-ERY PCR (AMOS is an acronym for B. abortus, B. melitensis, B. ovis and B. suis)), based on the multi-copy insertion element IS711 (also known as IS6501), is a multiplex assay that can differentiate B. abortus biovars 1, 2, 3b, 4, 5, 6 and 9 as well as the vaccine strains S19 and RB15. A PCR-RFLP assay based on the omp2 locus has been developed that differentiates B. abortus from other members of the genus, and when combined with RFLP can distinguish between biovars of B. abortus. Both the AMOS-ERY PCR and the PCR-RFLP methods have been widely adopted by the veterinary laboratories. Recently a Taqman real-time PCR assay using fluorogenic probes has been developed based on the sequence spanning the alkB gene and IS711. The real-time PCR assay has a detection threshold of 7.5 fg DNA (Bricker 2002; Michaux-Charachon et al. 1997; Moreno et al. 2002; Newby et al. 2003; Whatmore et al. 2005).

The 9 CFR 113.32: Detection of Brucella contamination describes the isolation of Brucella spp. in selective tryptose growth medium and detection of characteristic colonies. The 9 CFR 113.32 guidelines are not sufficiently specific or detailed, and the general method of culture isolation is not sufficiently sensitive for isolation of B. abortus.

The European Pharmacopoeia monographs Vaccines for veterinary use, 2.6.12 Microbiological examination of non-sterile products: microbial enumeration tests and 2.6.13 Microbiological examination of non-sterile products: test for specified microorganisms describe generalised methods for microbiological testing and selective methods of testing for specified microorganisms. The generalised methods described in the monograph 2.6.12 are not suitable for B. abortus detection. The monograph 2.6.13 does not include guidelines for B. abortus.

Brucella Canis

Culture isolation of Brucella canis can be performed on blood or on tryptose agar plates under aerobic conditions at 37 °C for 7 days (Keid et al. 2007). Initial inoculation of enrichment broth increases the success rate for culture isolation of B. canis.

Specific testing is recommended as bacteriological isolation is problematic and has a high rate of false negatives for B. canis.

A PCR assay has been developed for the 16S/23S rRNA interspace region that can detect as little as 3.8 fg of DNA. Systematic studies comparing PCR to culture isolation have shown that PCR has better sensitivity than culture isolation alone.

The 9 CFR 113.32: Detection of Brucella contamination describes the isolation of Brucella spp. in standard tryptose growth medium and detection of characteristic colonies. The 9 CFR 113.32 culture methods are problematic due to unacceptably high rates of false negatives and specific testing is required. The 9 CFR guidelines do not include specific testing for B. canis.

The European Pharmacopoeia monograph Vaccines for veterinary use, 2.6.12 Microbiological examination of non-sterile products: microbial enumeration tests and 2.6.13 Microbiological examination of non-sterile products: test for specified microorganisms describe generalised methods for microbiological testing and selective methods of testing for specified microorganisms. The generalised methods described in the monograph 2.6.12 are not suitable for B. canis detection. The monograph 2.6.13 does not include guidelines for B. canis.

Brucella Melitensis

Culture isolation of Brucella melitensis is possible on standard solid media such as tryptose agar under aerobic conditions at 37 °C. Additional isolation on the modified Thayer-Martin medium ensures detection of some strains of B. melitensis that are inhibited by nalidixic acid and bacitracin present in the Farrell's medium (Marin et al. 1996b; Marin et al. 1996a; Marín et al. 1999). Enrichment in broth culture prior to plating onto agar is recommended to enhance detection. Cultures should be maintained for 21 days and passaged at 7 day intervals to ensure detection. Cultures are incubated at 35 °C in 10 per cent CO2. Colony identification is by Gram-stained bacterial smears in which B. melitensis appears as small gram-negative coccobacilli. B. melitensis is positive for urea, catalase and oxidase in biochemical tests.

Specific testing is required for B. melitensis as low level detection is problematic even with the use of selective medium. Specific testing is possible by FA or PCR.

Confirmation of B. melitensis in bacterial smears is possible using specific reference antiserum in a FA.

PCR assays for B. melitensis have been developed targeting the 16S rRNA, bscp31 and IS 6501/ 711 molecular markers (Garin-Bastuji et al. 2006). Specific testing by real-time PCR targeting the IS711 gene can differentiate the 7 main clades or species of Brucella based on SNPs. Foster (2008) reports a detection threshold of 10 fg of DNA, detection sensitivity of 100 per cent and specificity of 100 per cent (Foster et al. 2008).

The 9 CFR 113.32: Detection of Brucella contamination describes the isolation of Brucella spp. in standard tryptose growth medium and detection of characteristic colonies. The 9 CFR 113.32 guidelines are not sufficiently specific or detailed, and the general method of culture isolation is not sufficiently sensitive for B. melitensis.

The European Pharmacopoeia monographs Vaccines for veterinary use, 2.6.12 Microbiological examination of non-sterile products: microbial enumeration tests and 2.6.13 Microbiological examination of non-sterile products: test for specified microorganisms describe generalised methods for microbiological testing and selective methods of testing for specified microorganisms. The generalised detection. The monograph 2.6.13 does not include guidelines for B. melitensis.

Brucella Suis

Brucella suis is cultured on enriched tryptic soy agar under aerobic conditions with 5 per cent CO_2. B. suis grows very slowly and cultures should be maintained for 4 weeks. On gram smears B. suis are gram-negative coccobacilli. Confirmation of B. suis is by slide-agglutination using anti-Brucella serum.

Genus specific PCR assays for Brucella have been developed targeting the OMP and 16S rRNA genes (Fekete et al. 1990; Romero et al. 1995) and genus specific probes have been used to differentiate Brucella spp. from Agrobacterium spp. (Fayazi et al. 2002; Herman and de Ridder 1992). A species specific PCR has been developed to differentiate Brucella abortus and Brucella suis based on the IS711 insertion sequence (Herman and de Ridder 1992). The PCR assay targeting the IS711 insertion sequence has been adapted to a real-time Taqman PCR assay using dual-labelled probes specific to B. melitensis, B. abortus and B. suis. The real-time Taqman PCR assay is highly sensitive, specific and accurate.

The 9 CFR 113.32: Detection of Brucella contamination protocol describes the isolation of Brucella spp. in selective tryptose growth medium and detection of characteristic colonies. The 9 CFR culture method describes optimal growth conditions for the culture isolation of B. suis. Confirmation of culture positives as B. suis would require specific testing.

The European Pharmacopoeia monographs Vaccines for veterinary use, 2.6.12 Microbiological examination of non-sterile products: microbial enumeration tests and 2.6.13 Microbiological examination of non-sterile products: test for specified microorganisms describe generalised methods for microbiological testing and selective methods of testing for specified microorganisms. The generalised methods described in the monograph 2.6.12 are not suitable for B. suis detection. The monograph 2.6.13 does not include guidelines for B. suis.

INFLUENZA A VIRUS SUBTYPE H5N1

Influenza A virus subtype H5N1, also known as A(H5N1) or simply H5N1, is a subtype of the influenza A virus which can cause illness in humans and many other animal species. A bird-adapted strain of H5N1, called HPAI A(H5N1) for highly pathogenic avian influenza virus of type A of subtype H5N1, is the highly pathogenic causative agent of H5N1 flu, commonly known as avian influenza ("bird flu").

It is enzootic in many bird populations, especially in Southeast Asia. One strain of HPAI A(H5N1) is spreading globally after first appearing in Asia. It is epizootic (an epidemic in nonhumans) and panzootic (affecting animals of and spurring the culling of hundreds of millions of others to stem its spread. Many references to "bird flu" and H5N1 in the popular media refer to this strain.

According to the World Health Organization and United Nations Food and Agriculture Organization, H5N1 pathogenicity is gradually continuing to rise in endemic areas, but the avian influenza disease situation in farmed birds is being held in check by vaccination, and so far there is "no evidence of sustained human-to-human transmission" of the virus. Eleven outbreaks of H5N1 were reported worldwide in June 2008 in five countries (China, Egypt, Indonesia, Pakistan and Vietnam) compared to 65 outbreaks in June 2006 and 55 in June 2007. The global HPAI situation significantly improved in the first half of 2008, but the FAO reports that imperfect disease surveillance systems mean that occurrence of the virus remains underestimated and underreported. In July 2013 the WHO announced a total of 630 confirmed human cases which resulted in the deaths of 375 people since 2003.

Several H5N1 vaccines have been developed and approved, and stockpiled by a number of countries, including the United States (in its National Stockpile), Britain, France, Canada, and Australia, for use in an emergency.

Research has shown that a highly contagious strain of H5N1, one that might allow airborne transmission between mammals, can be reached in only a few mutations, raising concerns about a pandemic and bioterrorism.

HPAI A(H5N1) is considered an avian disease, although there is some evidence of limited human-to-human transmission of the virus. A risk factor for contracting the virus is handling of infected poultry, but transmission of the virus from infected birds to humans has been characterized as inefficient. Still, around 60 per cent of humans known to have been infected with the current Asian strain of HPAI A(H5N1) have died from it, and H5N1 may mutate or reassort into a strain capable of efficient human-to-human transmission. In 2003, world-renowned virologist Robert G. Websterpublished an article titled "The world is teetering on the edge of a pandemic that could kill a large fraction of the human population" in American Scientist. He called for adequate resources to fight what he sees as a major world threat to possibly billions of lives.

On September 29, 2005,David Nabarro, the newly appointed Senior United Nations System Coordinator for Avian and Human Influenza, warned the world that an outbreak of avian influenza could kill anywhere between 5 million and 150 million people. Experts have identified key events (creating new clades, infecting new species, spreading to new areas) marking the progression of an avian flu virus towards becoming pandemic, and many of those key events have occurred more rapidly than expected.

Due to the high lethality and virulence of HPAI A(H5N1), its endemic presence, its increasingly large host reservoir, and its significant ongoing mutations, the H5N1 virus has recently been regarded to be the world's largest current pandemic threat, and billions of dollars are being spent researching H5N1 and preparing for a potential influenza pandemic. At least 12 companies and 17 governments are developing prepandemicinfluenza vaccines in 28 different clinical trials that, if successful, could turn a deadly pandemic infection into a non-deadly one. Full-scale production of a vaccine that could prevent any illness at all from the strain would require at least three months after the virus's emergence to begin, but it is hoped that vaccine production could increase until one billion doses were produced by one year after the initial identification of the virus.

H5N1 may cause more than one influenza pandemic, as it is expected to continue mutating in birds regardless of whether humans develop herd immunity to a future pandemic strain. Influenza pandemics from its genetic offspring may include influenza A virus subtypes other than H5N1. While genetic analysis of the H5N1 virus shows that influenza pandemics from its genetic offspring can easily be far more lethal than the Spanish flu pandemic, planning for a future influenza pandemic is based on what can be done and there is no higher Pandemic Severity Index level than a Category 5 pandemic which, roughly speaking, is any pandemic as bad as the Spanish flu or worse; and for which allintervention measures are to be used.

Signs and Symptoms

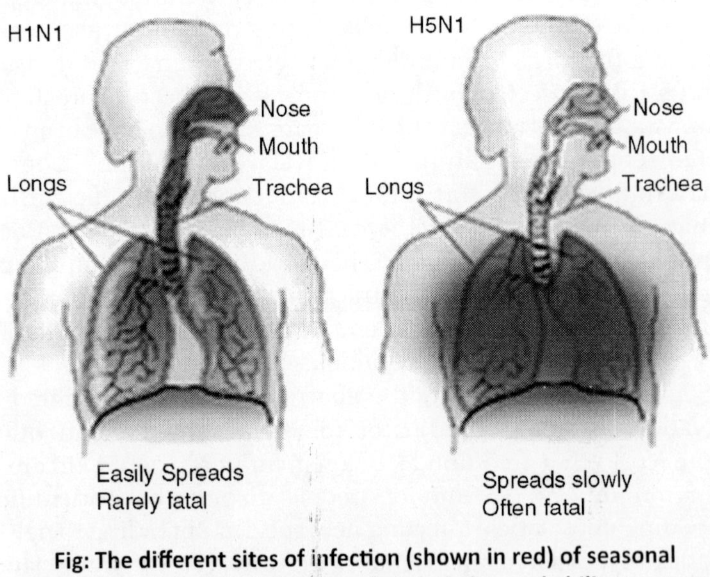

Fig: The different sites of infection (shown in red) of seasonal H1N1versus avian H5N1 influences their lethality and ability to spread.

The avian influenza hemagglutinin binds alpha 2-3 sialic acid receptors, while human influenza hemagglutinins bind alpha 2-6 sialic acid receptors. This means when the H5N1 strain infects humans, it will replicate in the lower respiratory tract, and consequently will causeviral pneumonia. There is as yet no human form of H5N1, so all humans who have caught it so far have caught avian H5N1. In general, humans who catch a humanized influenza A virus (a human flu virus of type A) usually have symptoms that include fever, cough, sore throat, muscle aches, conjunctivitis, and, in severe cases, breathing problems and pneumonia that may be fatal. The severity of the infection depends in large part on the state of the infected persons' immune systems and whether they had been exposed to the strain before (in which case they would be partially immune). No one knows if these or other symptoms will be the symptoms of a humanized H5N1 flu.

The reported mortality rate of highly pathogenic H5N1 avian influenza in a human is high; WHO data indicate 60 per cent of cases classified as H5N1 resulted in death. However, there is some evidence the actual mortality rate of avian flu could be much lower, as there may be many people with milder symptoms who do not seek treatment and are not counted.

In one case, a boy with H5N1 experienced diarrhea followed rapidly by a coma without developing respiratory or flu-like symptoms.There have been studies of the levels of cytokines in humans infected by the H5N1 flu virus. Of particular concern is elevated levels oftumor necrosis factor-alpha, a protein associated with tissue destruction at sites of infection and increased production of other cytokines. Flu virus-induced increases in the level of cytokines is also associated with flu symptoms, including fever, chills, vomiting and headache. Tissue damage associated with pathogenic flu virus infection can ultimately result in death. The inflammatory cascade triggered by H5N1 has been called a 'cytokine storm' by some, because of what seems to be a positive feedback process of damage to the body resulting from immune system stimulation. H5N1 induces higher levels of cytokines than the more common flu virus types.

Genetics

The first known strain of HPAI A(H5N1) (called A/chicken/Scotland/59) killed two flocks of chickens in Scotland in 1959, but that strain was very different from the current highly pathogenic strain of H5N1. The dominant strain of HPAI A(H5N1) in 2004 evolved from 1999 to 2002 creating the Z genotype. It has also been called "Asian lineage HPAI A(H5N1)".

Asian lineage HPAI A(H5N1) is divided into two antigenic clades. "Clade 1 includes human and bird isolates from Vietnam, Thailand, and Cambodiaand bird isolates from Laos and Malaysia. Clade 2 viruses were first identified in bird isolates from China, Indonesia, Japan, and South Koreabefore spreading westward to the Middle East, Europe, and Africa. The clade 2 viruses have been primarily responsible for human H5N1 infections that have occurred six subclades of clade 2, three of which have a distinct geographic distribution and have been implicated in human infections: Map

- Subclade 1, Indonesia
- Subclade 2, Europe, Middle East, and Africa (called EMA)
- Subclade 3, China"

A 2007 study focused on the EMA subclade has shed further light on the EMA mutations. "The 36 new isolates reported here greatly expand the amount of whole-genome sequence data available from recent avian influenza (H5N1) isolates. Before our project, GenBank contained only 5 other complete genomes from Europe for the 2004–2006 period, and it contained no whole genomes from the Middle East or northern Africa.

Our analysis showed several new findings. First, all European, Middle Eastern, and African samples fall into a clade that is distinct from other contemporary Asian clades, all of which share common ancestry with the original 1997 Hong Kong strain. Phylogenetic trees built on each of the 8 segments show a consistent picture of 3 lineages, as illustrated by the HA tree.

Two of the clades contain exclusively Vietnamese isolates; the smaller of these, with 5 isolates, we label V1; the larger clade, with 9 isolates, is V2. The remaining 22 isolates all fall into a third, clearly distinct clade, labeled EMA, which comprises samples from Europe, the Middle East, and Africa. Trees for the other 7 segments display a similar topology, with clades V1, V2, and EMA clearly separated in each case.

Analyses of all available complete influenza (H5N1) genomes and of 589 HA sequences placed the EMA clade as distinct from the major clades circulating in People's Republic of China, Indonesia, and Southeast Asia."

Terminology

H5N1 isolates are identified like this actual HPAI A(H5N1) example, A/chicken/Nakorn-Patom/Thailand/CU-K2/04(H5N1):

- A stands for the genus of influenza (A, B or C).
- Chicken is the animal species the isolate was found in (note: human isolates lack this component term and are thus identified as human isolates by default)
- Nakorn-Patom/Thailand is the place this specific virus was isolated
- CU-K2 is the laboratory reference number that identifies it from other influenza viruses isolated at the same place and year
- 04 Represents the year of isolation 2004
- H5 Stands for the fifth of several known types of the protein hemagglutinin.

- N 1 Stands for the first of several known types of the protein neuraminidase.

Other examples include: A/duck/Hong Kong/308/78(H5N3), A/avian/ NY/01(H5N2), A/chicken/Mexico/31381-3/94(H5N2), and A/shoveler/ Egypt/03(H5N2).

As with other avian flu viruses, H5N1 has strains called "highly pathogenic" (HP) and "low-pathogenic" (LP). Avian influenza viruses that cause HPAI are highly virulent, and mortality rates in infected flocks often approach 100 per cent. LPAI viruses have negligible virulence, but these viruses can serve as progenitors to HPAI viruses. The current strain of H5N1 responsible for the deaths of birds across the world is an HPAI strain; all other current strains of H5N1, including a North American strain that causes no disease at all in any species, are LPAI strains. All HPAI strains identified to date have involved H5 and H7 subtypes. The distinction concerns pathogenicity in poultry, not humans. Normally, a highly pathogenic avian virus is not highly pathogenic to either humans or non-poultry birds. This current deadly strain of H5N1 is unusual in being deadly to so many species, including some, like domestic cats, never previously susceptible to any influenza virus.

Genetic Structure and Related Subtypes

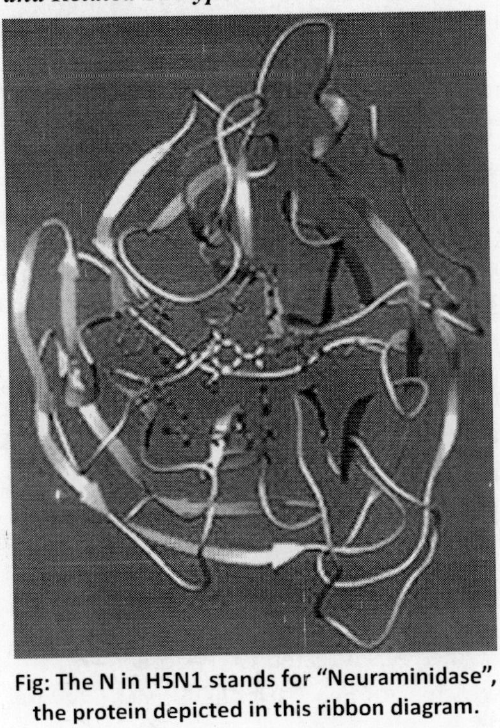

Fig: The N in H5N1 stands for "Neuraminidase", the protein depicted in this ribbon diagram.

H5N1 is a subtype of the species Influenza A virus of the Influenzavirus A genus of the Orthomyxoviridae family. Like all other influenza A subtypes, the H5N1 subtype is an RNA virus. It has a segmented genome of eight negative sense, single-strands of RNA, abbreviated as PB2, PB1, PA, HA, NP, NA, MP and NS.

HA codes for hemagglutinin, an antigenic glycoprotein found on the surface of the influenza viruses and is responsible for binding the virus to the cell that is being infected. NA codes for neuraminidase, an antigenic glycosylated enzyme found on the surface of the influenza viruses. It facilitates the release of progeny viruses from infected cells. The hemagglutinin (HA) and neuraminidase (NA) RNA strands specify the structure of proteins that are most medically relevant as targets for antiviral drugs and antibodies. HA and NA are also used as the basis for the naming of the different subtypes of influenza A viruses. This is where the H and N come from in H5N1.

Influenza A viruses are significant for their potential for disease and death in humans and other animals. Influenza A virus subtypes that have been confirmed in humans, in order of the number of known human pandemic deaths that they have caused, include:

- H1N1, which caused the 1918 flu pandemic ("Spanish flu") and currently is causing seasonal human flu and the 2009 flu pandemic ("swine flu")
- H2N2, which caused "Asian flu"
- H3N2, which caused "Hong Kong flu" and currently causes seasonal human flu
- H5N1, ("bird flu"), which is noted for having a strain (Asian-lineage HPAI H5N1) that kills over half the humans it infects, infecting and killing species that were never known to suffer from influenza viruses before (e.g. cats), being unable to be stopped by culling all involved poultry - some think due to being endemic in wild birds, and causing billions of dollars to be spent in flu pandemic preparation and preventiveness
- H7N7, which has unusual zoonotic potential and killed one person
- H1N2, which is currently endemic in humans and pigs and causes seasonal human flu
- H9N2, which has infected three people
- H7N2, which has infected two people
- H7N3, which has infected two people
- H10N7, which has infected two people
- H7N9, which as of Feb 2014 has infected 309 people, and lead to 70 deaths

Low pathogenic H5N1

Low pathogenic avian influenza H5N1 (LPAI H5N1) also called "North American" H5N1 commonly occurs in wild birds. In most cases, it causes minor sickness or no noticeable signs of disease in birds. It is not known to affect humans at all. The only concern about it is that it is possible for it to be transmitted to poultry and in poultry mutate into a highly pathogenic strain.

- 1966 - LPAI H5N1 A/Turkey/Ontario/6613/1966(H5N1) was detected in a flock of infected turkeys in Ontario, Canada
- 1975 – LPAI H5N1 was detected in a wild mallard duck and a wild blue goose in Wisconsin.
- 1981 and 1985 – LPAI H5N1 was detected in ducks by the University of Minnesota conducting a sampling procedure in which sentinel ducks were monitored in cages placed in the wild for a short period of time.
- 1983 – LPAI H5N1 was detected in ring-billed gulls in Pennsylvania.
- 1986 - LPAI H5N1 was detected in a wild mallard duck in Ohio.
- 2005 - LPAI H5N1 was detected in ducks in Manitoba, Canada.
- 2008 - LPAI H5N1 was detected in ducks in New Zealand.
- 2009 - LPAI H5N1 was detected in commercial poultry in British Columbia.

"In the past, there was no requirement for reporting or tracking LPAI H5 or H7 detections in wild birds so states and universities tested wild bird samples independently of USDA. Because of this, the above list of previous detections might not be all inclusive of past LPAI H5N1 detections. However, the World Organization for Animal Health (OIE) recently changed its requirement of reporting detections of avian influenza. Effective in 2006, all confirmed LPAI H5 and H7 AI subtypes must be reported to the OIE because of their potential to mutate into highly pathogenic strains. Therefore, USDA now tracks these detections in wild birds, backyard flocks, commercial flocks and live bird markets."

High Mutation Rate

Influenza viruses have a relatively high mutation rate that is characteristic of RNA viruses. The segmentation of its genome facilitates genetic recombination by segmentreassortment in hosts infected with two different influenza viruses at the same time. A previously uncontagious strain may then be able to pass between humans, one of several possible paths to a pandemic.

The ability of various influenza strains to show species-selectivity is largely due to variation in the hemagglutinin genes. Genetic mutations in the hemagglutinin gene that cause single amino acid substitutions can significantly alter the ability of viral hemagglutinin proteins to bind to receptors on the surface of host cells.

Such mutations in avian H5N1 viruses can change virus strains from being inefficient at infecting human cells to being as efficient in causing human infections as more common human influenza virus types.This doesn't mean that one amino acid substitution can cause a pandemic, but it does mean that one amino acid substitution can cause an avian flu virus that is not pathogenic in humans to become pathogenic in humans.

Influenza A virus subtype H3N2 is endemic in pigs in China, and has been detected in pigs in Vietnam, increasing fears of the emergence of new variant strains. The dominant strain of annual flu virus in January 2006 was H3N2, which is now resistant to the standard antiviral drugs amantadine and rimantadine. The possibility of H5N1 and H3N2 exchanging genes through reassortment is a major concern. If a reassortment in H5N1 occurs, it might remain an H5N1 subtype, or it could shift subtypes, as H2N2 did when it evolved into the Hong Kong Flu strain of H3N2.

Both the H2N2 and H3N2 pandemic strains contained avian influenza virus RNA segments. "While the pandemic human influenza viruses of 1957 (H2N2) and 1968 (H3N2) clearly arose through reassortment between human and avian viruses, the influenza virus causing the 'Spanish flu' in 1918 appears to be entirely derived from an avian source".

Prevention

Vaccine: There are several H5N1 vaccines for several of the avian H5N1 varieties, but the continual mutation of H5N1 renders them of limited use to date: while vaccines can sometimes provide cross-protection against related flu strains, the best protection would be from a vaccine specifically produced for any future pandemic flu virus strain. Dr. Daniel Lucey, co-director of the Biohazardous Threats and Emerging Diseases graduate programme at Georgetown University has made this point, "There is no H5N1 pandemic so there can be no pandemic vaccine". However, "pre-pandemic vaccines" have been created; are being refined and tested; and do have some promise both in furthering research and preparedness for the next pandemic. Vaccine manufacturing companies are being encouraged to increase capacity so that if a pandemic vaccine is needed, facilities will be available for rapid production of large amounts of a vaccine specific to a new pandemic strain.

Public Health

"The United States is collaborating closely with eight international organizations, including the World Health Organization (WHO), the Food and Agriculture Organization of the United Nations (FAO), the World Organization for Animal Health (OIE), and 88 foreign governments to address the situation through planning, greater monitoring, and full transparency in reporting and investigating avian influenza occurrences.

The United States and these international partners have led global efforts to encourage countries to heighten surveillance for outbreaks in poultry and significant numbers of deaths in migratory birds and to rapidly introduce containment measures. The U.S. Agency for International Development (USAID) and the U.S. Department of State, the U.S. Department of Health and Human Services (HHS), and Agriculture (USDA) are coordinating future international response measures on behalf of the White House with departments and agencies across the federal government".

Together steps are being taken to "minimize the risk of further spread in animal populations", "reduce the risk of human infections", and "further support pandemic planning and preparedness".

Ongoing detailed mutually coordinated onsite surveillance and analysis of human and animal H5N1 avian flu outbreaks are being conducted and reported by the USGS National Wildlife Health Center, the Centers for Disease Control and Prevention, the World Health Organization, the European Commission, and others.

Treatment

There is no highly effective treatment for H5N1 flu, but oseltamivir (commercially marketed by Roche as Tamiflu), can sometimes inhibit the influenza virus from spreading inside the user's body. This drug has become a focus for some governments and organizations trying to prepare for a possible H5N1 pandemic. On April 20, 2006, Roche AG announced that a stockpile of three million treatment courses of Tamiflu are waiting at the disposal of the World Health Organization to be used in case of a flu pandemic; separately Roche donated two million courses to the WHO for use in developing nations that may be affected by such a pandemic but lack the ability to purchase large quantities of the drug.

However, WHO expert Hassan al-Bushra has said:

"Even now, we remain unsure about Tamiflu's real effectiveness. As for a vaccine, work cannot start on it until the emergence of a new virus, and we predict it would take six to nine months to develop it. For the moment, we cannot by any means count on a potential vaccine to prevent the spread of a contagious influenza virus, whose various precedents in the past 90 years have been highly pathogenic".

Animal and lab studies suggest that Relenza (zanamivir), which is in the same class of drugs as Tamiflu, may also be effective against H5N1. In a study performed on mice in 2000, "zanamivir was shown to be efficacious in treating avian influenza viruses H9N2, H6N1, and H5N1 transmissible to mammals". In addition, mice studies suggest the combination of zanamivir, celecoxib and mesalazine looks promising producing a 50 per cent survival rate compared to no survival in the placebo arm. While no one knows if zanamivir will be useful or not on a yet to exist pandemic strain of H5N1, it an H5N1 influenza pandemic. Neither oseltamivir nor zanamivir can currently be manufactured in quantities that would be meaningful once efficient human transmission starts. In September, 2006, a WHO scientist announced that studies had confirmed cases of H5N1 strains resistant to Tamiflu and Amantadine. Tamiflu-resistant strains have also appeared in the EU, which remain sensitive to Relenza.

Epidemiology

The earliest infections of humans by H5N1 coincided with an epizootic (an epidemic in non-humans) of H5N1 influenza in Hong Kong's poultry population. This panzootic (a disease affecting animals of many species, especially over a wide area) outbreak was stopped by the killing of the entire domestic poultry population within the territory. However, the disease has continued to spread. On December 21, 2009 the WHO announced a total of 447 cases which resulted in the deaths of 263.

Contagiousness

H5N1 is easily transmissible between birds, facilitating a potential global spread of H5N1. While H5N1 undergoes mutation and reassortment, creating variations which can infect species not previously known to carry the virus, not all of these variant forms can infect humans. H5N1 as an avian virus preferentially binds to a type of galactose receptors that populate the avian respiratory tract from the nose to the lungs and are virtually absent in humans, occurring only in and around the alveoli, structures deep in the lungs where oxygen is passed to the blood. Therefore, the virus is not easily expelled by coughing and sneezing, the usual route of transmission.

H5N1 is mainly spread by domestic poultry, both through the movements of infected birds and poultry products and through the use of infected poultry manure as fertilizer or feed. Humans with H5N1 have typically caught it from chickens, which were in turn infected by other poultry or waterfowl. Migrating waterfowl (wild ducks, geese and swans) carry H5N1, often without becoming sick. Many species of birds and mammals can be infected with HPAI A(H5N1), but the role of animals other than poultry and waterfowl as disease- spreading hosts is unknown.

According to a report by the World Health Organization, H5N1 may be spread indirectly. The report stated the virus may sometimes stick to surfaces or get kicked up in fertilizer dust to infect people.

Virulence

H5N1 has mutated into a variety of strains with differing pathogenic profiles, some pathogenic to one species but not others, some pathogenic to multiple species. Each specific known genetic variation is traceable to a virus isolate of a specific case of infection. Through antigenic drift, H5N1 has mutated into dozens of highly pathogenic varieties divided into genetic clades which are known from specific isolates, but all currently belonging to genotype Z of avian influenza virus H5N1, now the dominant genotype. H5N1 isolates found in Hong Kong in 1997 and 2001 were not consistently transmitted efficiently among birds and did not cause significant disease in these animals. In 2002, new isolates of H5N1 were appearing within the bird population of Hong Kong. These new isolates caused acute disease, including severe neurological dysfunction and death inducks. This was the first reported case of lethal influenza virus infection in wild aquatic birds since 1961. Genotype Z emerged in 2002 through reassortment from earlier highly pathogenic genotypes of H5N1 that first infected birds in China in 1996, and first infected humans in Hong Kong in 1997. Genotype Z is endemic in birds in Southeast Asia, has created at least two clades that can infect humans, and is spreading across the globe in bird populations. Mutations occurring within this genotype are increasing their pathogenicity. Birds are also able to shed the virus for longer periods of time before their death, increasing the transmissibility of the virus.

Transmission and Host Range

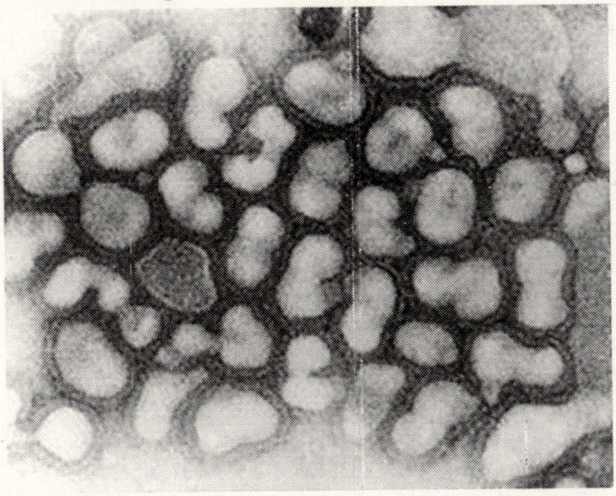

Fig: Influenza A virus is the virus that causes avian flu:

Transmission electron micrograph of negatively stained virus particles in late passage.

Infected birds transmit H5N1 through their saliva, nasal secretions, feces and blood. Other animals may become infected with the virus through direct contact with these bodily fluids or through contact with surfaces contaminated with them. H5N1 remains infectious after over 30 days at 0°C (32.0°F) (over one month at freezing temperature) or 6 days at 37°C (98.6°F) (one week at human body temperature); at ordinary temperatures it lasts in the environment for weeks. In Arctic temperatures, it does not degrade at all.

H5N1 virus, it is spreading to all parts of the world. H5N1 is different from all previously known highly pathogenic avian flu viruses in its ability to be spread by animals other than poultry.

In October 2004, researchers discovered H5N1 is far more dangerous than was previously believed. Waterfowl were revealed to be directly spreading this highly pathogenic strain to chickens, crows, pigeons, and other birds, and the virus was increasing its ability to infect mammals, as well. From this point on, avian flu experts increasingly referred to containment as a strategy that can delay, but not ultimately prevent, a future avian flu pandemic.

"Since 1997, studies of influenza A (H5N1) indicate that these viruses continue to evolve, with changes in antigenicity and internal gene constellations; an expanded host range in avian species and the ability to infect felids; enhanced pathogenicity in experimentally infected mice and ferrets, in which they cause systemic infections; and increased environmental stability."

The New York Times, in an article on transmission of H5N1 through smuggled birds, reports Wade Hagemeijer of Wetlands International stating, "We believe it is spread by both bird migration and trade, but that trade, particularly illegal trade, is more important".

□

Index

□□□